Higher Education
for
Public Health

Higher Education
for
Public Health

A REPORT OF
THE MILBANK MEMORIAL FUND COMMISSION

CECIL G. SHEPS, CHAIRMAN

Published for the Milbank Memorial Fund by
PRODIST
New York   •   1976

Published for the
Milbank Memorial Fund
by
PRODIST
a division of
Neale Watson Academic Publications, Inc.
156 Fifth Avenue, New York, N.Y. 10010

Library of Congress Cataloging in Publication Data

Milbank Memorial Fund.   Commission.
   Higher education for public health.

   Bibliography: p.
   1.   Public health—Study and teaching—United States.
I.   Sheps, Cecil George, 1913–   II.   Title.   [DNLM:
1.   Public health—Education.   WA18 M638h]
RA440.6.M55   1976   362.1'07'1173   76–6951
ISBN 0–88202–065–X

Designed and manufactured in the U.S.A.

Contents

Foreword

Sixty years ago, when the Johns Hopkins University established the first school of public health, it marked a turning point in public health education. Specialization in public health was a new concept and the School was to be an institute for research and training in the science of hygiene and public health, and its application. The research emphasis and the essential relationship with other schools and disciplines of the university introduced a new model and new standards for the teaching and practice of public health.

The enactment of the Social Security Act in 1935 provided a major impetus to public health education, stimulating the development of several new schools and an increase in the enrollment of existing schools. Today there are 20 schools of public health in both private and public universities in the United States. They have served with distinction as a national and international resource for the education of health manpower, and their impact has been manifold, not only upon the practice of public health but also upon its conceptual relation to broader social issues.

In recent years, there has developed an increasing skepticism of higher education, its relevance, effectiveness, and benefits. This skepticism extended to education for the health professions, including, but not limited to, schools of public health.

Questions are being asked as to the presumed relationship between professional education and professional practice. Is there a profound distinction between traditional educational norms and standards, and the rapidly changing role models for which education was undertaken? If so, shall emphasis for change be on educational input or the practice model?

What is the role of medical schools and their departments of community medicine? Can they perform some of the functions of a school of public health or is their potential contribution seriously constrained because of their emphasis upon education for treatment of the sick and the dominance of the clinical faculty in teaching and investigation? Have schools of public health, like medical schools, become so dependent upon federal funds that their policies and programs are determined by dollars available and they no longer control their own destiny?

Schools of public health were cognizant of these questions and recognized that in addition to changing health problems and needs, social, economic, and political changes were occurring. They were cognizant, too, of the increasing contributions and functions of the total university in education for public health.

In 1971, the Association of Schools of Public Health requested the Milbank Memorial Fund to organize and support a study of the role of universities in higher education for public health. The staff of the Fund discussed the proposal with a number of university officials, practitioners in public health, and staff of the Public Health Service, and were encouraged to support such a study.

Accordingly, a Commission was established by the Fund in 1972. We were fortunate that Dr. Cecil G. Sheps accepted our invitation to chair the Commission and assume major responsibility for the selection of distinguished Commission members who might represent the health professions, disciplines cognate to public health, higher education, and the public interest. Funding for three years was provided.

The Milbank Memorial Fund Commission for the Study of Higher Education for Public Health was organizationally and administratively separate from the Fund and had complete freedom and autonomy in planning and executing its activities and in making its recommendations. The charge to the Commission by the Fund was to execute a comprehensive study of higher education for public health in universities, with major emphasis upon schools of public health, in order to help develop a new unity of purpose and direction as these institutions attempt to respond to profound changes in values, expectations, and needs of society.

Just as the first school of public health revolutionized the concept of the scientific knowledge base and teaching methods in public health, so it is hoped that the report of this study and its recommendations will assist higher education for public health to respond effectively and adapt to new directions and changing needs.

The fact that changes have occurred even within the four years since this study was initiated indicates that more important than a set of solutions may be the evolution of a continuing process of monitoring change and creating ever-new and elastic responses which meet the needs of society and at the same time safeguard elements of proven excellence.

The Milbank Memorial Fund has been happy to support this program. The Fund, established in 1905, has been primarily identified with, and involved in, public health. We commend highly the sincere interest, earnest commitment, and serious efforts of the Chairman and distinguished Commission members. We also wish to extend our grateful thanks and appreciation to Dr. Florence Kavaler, Study Director, who has since accepted a commission in the Public Health Service.

The report will not satisfy everyone nor answer all the questions. It will have a positive impact, however, if it exposes the major issues and if it promotes discussion, debate, and controversy.

L.E. BURNEY

PRESIDENT

MILBANK MEMORIAL FUND

Milbank Memorial Fund Commission
for the Study of Higher Education
for Public Health

Frederick C. Robbins
Dean
School of Medicine
Case Western Reserve University
Cleveland, Ohio

Charles L. Schottland
Professor of Social Welfare
Florence Heller Graduate School for
   Advanced Studies in Social Welfare
Brandeis University
Waltham, Massachusetts

George A. Silver
Professor of Public Health
Department of Epidemiology
   and Public Health
Yale University
School of Medicine
New Haven, Connecticut

Study Director
Florence Kavaler

Editorial Consultant
Marjorie Taubenhaus

Acknowledgments

The Commission conducted its work largely in the form of a committee of the whole, although it did, on occasion, delegate certain investigative and consultative activities to one or more of its members. Its work was greatly assisted by data, views, and advice provided by many consultants who came from all areas of public health practice and education, from several levels of government, and from individuals concerned with national health policy and university administration. The Commission wishes to express its thanks to them for giving so generously of their experience, interest, and time.

Such contributions were made from the field of public health education by Dr. Charles Austin, Dr. Lester Breslow, Dr. Donald A. Cornely, Mr. Raymond D. Colton, Dr. William A. Darity, Dr. Robert W. Day, Dr. Chester W. Douglass, Dr. Gary L. Filerman, Dr. Ruth B. Freeman, Dr. Bernard G. Greenberg, Dr. Herschel E. Griffin, Dr. Thomas Hall, Ms. Effie S. Hanchett, Mr. Nathan Hershey, Dr. John C. Hume, Dr. B. Jon Jaeger, Dr. Anthony R. Kovner, Dr. Lowell Levin, Dr. Stanley Mayers, Dr. Fred Mayes, Ms. Virginia Nelson, Dr. Daniel Okun, Dr. Virginia Maye Ohlson, Dr. Paul Q. Peterson, Dr. Harry Phillips, Dr. Leonard S. Rosenfeld, Dr. Morris Schaeffer, Dr. Conrad Seipp, Dr. Margaret L. Shetland, Dr. Reuel A. Stallones, Dr. James H. Sterner, Dr. Guy W. Steuart, Ms. Janet A. Strauss, Dr. Carl E. Taylor, Dr. Myron Wegman, Dr. Kerr L. White, and Dr. Byron Wight.

From the field of public health practice, we were assisted by Mr. Stephen J. Ackerman, Dr. John Atwater, Dr. E. Kenneth Aycock, Dr. Jack Butler, Dr. Paul B. Cornely, Ms. Joan S. Davis, Dr. Kenneth M. Endicott, Dr. Leonard D. Fenninger, Mr. Larry Gordon, Dr. Walter Hoover, Ms. Robah Kellogg, Dr. Stephen H. King, Dr. Jacob Koomen, Dr. Milo D. Leavitt, Dr. Fred McCrumb, Dr. Mary C. McLaughlin, Dr. Vaun A. Newill, Dr. Fred J. Payne, Dr. Donald M. Pitcairn, Dr. David P. Rall, Ms. Eva Reese, Dr. Milton S. Saslaw, Ms. Jessie M. Scott, Dr. Mack Shanholtz, Dr. Irving Shapiro, Dr.

Jerry Solon, Dr. William R. Stinger, Dr. Vernon E. Wilson, and Mr. Irwin Woikstein.

From the fields of higher education for related professions, and from university administration, we were helped by Dr. Ralph Boatman, Dr. John C. Beck, Dr. John Z. Bowers, Dr. Frederic Cleaveland, Dr. Kurt Deuschle, Dr. James Dixon, Dr. John R. Evans, Dr. Amasa B. Ford, Dr. J. Thomas Grayston, Dr. John H. Knowles, Dr. Lyle V. Jones, Dr. Moses S. Koch, Dr. Kenneth E. Penrod, Dr. George G. Reader, Dr. Sidney Rodenberg, Dr. David E. Rogers, Mr. Kenneth G. Skaggs, Dr. Emanuel Suter, Dr. Morton Teicher, Dr. Milton Terris, and Dr. Roman Villareal.

Others who assisted were Mr. Jay Constantine, Ms. Lynn Clark, Ms. Martha Clinton, Mr. Paul Danaceau, Mr. Ronald Ferrucci, Mrs. Ruth Hanft, Dr. Charlotte Muller, and Dr. Donald Ware.

We are especially grateful to colleagues in the United Kingdom and the World Health Organization who were good enough to consult with the Chairman: Dr. Brian Abel-Smith, Dr. John H. F. Brotherston, Dr. T. Fülöp, Dr. Walter W. Holland, Dr. Robert H. Hunter, Dr. Halfdan T. Mahler, Dr. Thomas McKeown, Mr. Gordon McLachlan, Dr. Alfonso Mejia, Dr. J.N. Morris, Dr. Kenneth Newell, Dr. John J.A. Reid, and Dr. Michael D. Warren.

During the third and last year of its work, the Commission arranged a series of informal meetings with selected groups of people because of its interest in their perceptions of the relevance and validity of the recommendations being developed. The Commission found these sessions especially helpful, and is deeply indebted to those who participated in them. There were nine such meetings with representatives from the Association of State and Territorial Health Officers, Department of Health, Education, and Welfare staff members, staff members of relevant congressional committees, the American Public Health Association, the Association of Academic Health Centers, the Association of Schools of Public Health, the Association of University Programs in Health Administration, the faculty of the Johns Hopkins School of Hygiene and Public Health, the Directors of Maternal and Child Health Programs in Schools of Public Health, the Association of Teachers of Preventive Medicine, the American Board of Preventive Medicine, and the American College of Preventive Medicine.

Introduction

The challenge of protecting and restoring the health of the American people appears ever more prominent on the agenda of our nation's domestic business. The United States' Congress is wrestling with numerous proposals for national health insurance while it debates the use of the increasing billions of dollars which it appropriates for medical care. State legislatures are finding the rising costs of the state share of Medicaid inimical to a balanced budget and are cutting funds for these and other health programs. Each day a newspaper headline warns of threats to life and health: the Food and Drug Administration bans the use of yet another food additive, lethal gas freed in oil-gas production poses an increasing hazard, and even drugs prescribed for the relief of suffering are found to be dangerous to human health.

Most people believe that the way to improve health is through more medical care, more doctors, and more hospitals. They are beginning to realize, however, that there are limits to what medical care can achieve. The United States spends more money on medical care (both absolutely and in relation to population) than any other country in the world, but most of the Western European nations have a lower infant mortality rate than ours and many have a longer average life expectancy.

This does not mean that we should not improve medical care. At present, poor people and rural people do not have ready access to it, its cost rising sharply, and its quality is too often questionable. The task of reshaping our massive, pluralistic medical care system is urgent, but it must be undertaken in conjunction with a total community perspective which gives equal attention to other types of activities to protect health and prevent disease.

The limits to possible health achievements through medical care are highlighted by the growing number of elements in our physical and social environment which are hazardous to health. While the traditional concerns of sanitary engineering are by no means handled adequately for the entire population, we are faced with yet new problems which require better methods than we now have to ensure that our food, drugs, water supply, and the air we breathe are safe and uncontaminated. Certain environmental hazards affect only those in particular occupations, but there are others which affect large sections of our population. Most of the hazards which are external to the human body are those which the individual or the medical care system do not, or cannot, control. The solution of these problems goes directly to the heart of the social and economic policies of our nation.

The emergence of chronic illness as a predominant health problem has produced a greater awareness of the major role in health of the habits and attitudes of individuals and groups, whole communities and, in some instances, the nation. The role of life-style in producing self-imposed risks, or in obstructing the implementation of measures which will reduce risk or facilitate the effectiveness of treatment, is increasingly being recognized. Alcohol addiction, cigarette smoking, the abuse of pharmaceuticals leading to drug dependence, improper diet, lack of exercise, and careless driving are all major problems whose solution depends upon changes in the life-style of individuals, communities, and the nation.

Before any substantial progress can be made, however, the public and its leaders must be able to make free decisions based upon full and valid information regarding the nature of health issues, the social policy needed to deal with them, and the kinds of programs and services which will best implement desired policies. For this to take place, we must have professional and technical personnel with adequate training and in appropriate numbers.

The Milbank Memorial Fund Commission for the Study of Higher Education for Public Health identified these background factors as crucial to an assessment of public health today, as it tried to distinguish those issues in public health that will demand attention tomorrow, to weigh the need for various types of professional personnel, and to evaluate the present efforts of our universities in higher education for public health. While it would be misleading to suggest that our universities are responsible for the defects and inadequacies in our national effort to solve health problems, these defects pose a great challenge to the universities. These institutions have the responsibility of educating people who must understand the important health issues, and lead and organize service programs to deal with them. The Milbank Memorial Fund Commission felt that its own contribution could best be made by posing the question: "How can the public health education programs of our universities make their most significant contribution to improving the health of the American people?" This led us to develop recommendations for the reorganization and systematization of the diverse programs, so that they would be more effective than the current efforts.

As with other health professions, there is currently much dissatisfaction with the training and abilities of personnel in public health, particularly those in leadership positions. In addition, there are substantial manpower shortages in certain fields. Serious criticisms of the various types of graduate programs come from many quarters. State health officers, directors of large health organizations (which are quasipublic), and members of the top echelon of the federal government complain that they have great difficulty finding professional personnel with appropriate skills and knowledge to meet the challenge of today's public health problems. Leading federal health officials have expressed doubt about the wisdom of the federal government moving into new areas and enlarging its programs because it is difficult to find professional personnel with the kind of preparation needed to deal effectively with the new challenges.

Faculty members in the schools of public health also express dismay and concern. Some of them find, for example, that they are hampered in providing advanced-level teaching when they face classes containing people from a wide range of backgrounds with widely varying levels of preparation. Not uncommonly, they meet classes that include physicians, engineers, nurses, and holders of graduate degrees in chemistry, biology, or sociology—some of whom have already had field experience in public health—along with students who have just obtained their baccalaureate degrees and have had no relevant field experience. Thus the faculty member is forced to scale down the level of his presentation to the lowest common denominator. Some students complain because they are getting material for which they lack adequate preparation or, more commonly, students with substantial preparation find that some course material is not challenging because it is aimed at the unprepared student.

Additionally, there is the criticism that schools of public health are training people for programs of the past and not for the future, and indeed may be incapable of making the changes that are needed. There are complaints that graduate programs in hospital or health administration in schools of business concentrate too heavily on the business aspects, and do not give adequate attention to the health objectives of the programs for which they are training administrators. This leads to the conclusion that there is confusion and lack of clarity about the objectives and purposes of current training programs for responsibilities in public health, and that inadequate attention has been given to the range of skills and knowledge now needed. There is a growing feeling that entirely new programs need to be developed, especially to prepare leadership personnel.

In view of the above, and also because of the great expansion in the scope of public health problems and the considerable growth of public programs, it seemed appropriate to the Milbank Memorial Fund that an appraisal be made of the current programs of education for this field in terms of their adequacy and potential for meeting the needs of this enlarging area of human service.

In the past decade in the United States, higher education and education for the health professions have been the subject of a series of self-study efforts, task forces, and commissions. This has resulted in a number of reports devoted specifically to the problems of education for public health. In one way or another, all these reports are an outgrowth of dissatisfactions with existing programs, and reflect the growing demand for universities to become more responsive as institutions which serve society and facilitate change.

In 1966 the National Commission on Community Health Services produced a report which dealt, inter alia, with health manpower, the recruitment of students for health careers, and training for such careers. In 1967 the revised version of the final report of the Joint

Committee on the Study of Education for Public Health was issued. This committee was composed of representatives from the American Public Health Association, the Association of Schools of Public Health, and the Association of State and Territorial Health Officers. More recently, the W.K. Kellogg Foundation established an interdisciplinary Commission on Education for Health Administration, whose report was published in 1975.

The Milbank Memorial Fund Commission for the Study of Higher Education for Public Health grew out of a request made by the deans of schools of public health for a survey of their programs. The mandate of the Commission included not only these schools but all programs of higher education for public health in this country.

As the Commission reviewed thousands of pages of reports, literature, and consultants' staff and Commission members' memoranda and papers, a central theme developed: convinced that the public health movement's contribution to the health of Americans will depend to a great extent on the leadership of the public health programs and services, how can we best train such leadership?

This report is an attempt to contribute a point of view, ideas, and specific recommendations to accomplish this objective. In setting forth our views, we recognize that we have not been able to conduct a scientific study in the usual sense of that term. But the Commission members brought knowledge and experience from public administration, social policy analysis and development, higher education administration, public health administration, public health education, environmental health, medical education, and social service administration, practice, and education to our considerations and study. Representing different disciplines and various points of view, the Commission evolved a set of recommendations upon which there was agreement—recommendations which we believe will enable our universities to make their most effective contribution to public health.

We are not suggesting that technology and managerial skill will solve all the health problems of our nation. Health policy issues must first be addressed effectively. American health policy is clouded in conflicts over basic social values. While access to health care is widely proclaimed as a "right," political and economic policy decisions frequently confound that assertion and reflect the basic ambivalence which characterizes the history of American social policy. As these issues become more complex, more expertise is needed. We believe that our nation will be able to grapple with health and economic issues more clearly and directly if it can benefit from the highest quality professional efforts to uncover, assemble, and synthesize relevant information and to develop the best measures to deal with the problems. Thus a high level of professional performance in public health is a pressing social necessity. It is crucial that educational programs for this purpose be of the highest possible quality.

We hope our report will help those who are concerned with the conduct and support of higher education to clarify the mission they might wish to fulfill in public health. We also hope that it will help the leaders of public health agencies to compare the different types of educational programs to see which best serve their employment needs.

We recognize that the recommendations that we have made are not the only possible ones. We hope, however, that our review of needs and current efforts and our delineation of pathways toward a more rational framework for all the efforts in higher education for public health will provoke further open-minded, vigorous, and innovative consideration of policies and actions which will lead to an increase in the professional effectiveness of those who work in the field.

I: The Field
of Public Health

1. Public Health Defined

Public health is the effort organized by society to protect, promote, and restore the people's health. The programs, services, and institutions involved emphasize the prevention of disease and the health needs of the population as a whole. Public health activities change with changing technology and social values, but the goals remain the same: to reduce the amount of disease, premature death, and disease-produced discomfort and disability.

This definition was developed by the Commission in order to delineate the field to which higher education for public health must address itself. We felt that the definition must be narrow enough to be made operational and yet broad enough to encompass all the activities and personnel now considered in the sphere of public health. For this reason, we have emphasized the organized nature of the effort involved, as well as the community, public, and preventive aspects essential to public health.

The Commission emphasizes "organized efforts" because there are many elements in American society today which have the protection or promotion of health as their primary objective, or which contribute secondarily to these goals. Examples abound, such as physicians in private practice or companies manufacturing drugs. But these, as do many others, function on an individual, almost entrepreneurial basis and participate only peripherally in planned programs for the promotion or restoration of health. As such, they would not be considered as part of public health, although their contributions are essential to the success of the total effort.

Instead of considering health problems simply as they occur in a series of individuals, the public health perspective views these same problems in the context of the community as a whole. This permits the establishment of priorities, and allows rational choices to be made about the use of resources. The community perspective is also the only one which permits identification of what is not being accomplished as well as what is.

There is also a commitment in public health concerns and activities to be of a communal rather than a personal nature. This makes possible the solution of community-wide problems, as it is rare for any element in the private sector to have the power, resources, or motivation that official government agencies possess. This perspective does not depreciate the dignity and importance of the individual, but rather emphasizes the cogency of the broad view so that society's resources can be allocated to benefit the health of the population as a whole.

Public Standards

One traditional way for the community view to be enforced is through the application of public standards for products and performance. These standards are applied in health fields and many other situations where life and health may be at stake, in order to ensure competence and quality and protect against health hazards.

Public standards are also an example of the traditional public health emphasis on prevention of disease and disability, as distinct from medical practice which emphasizes curing or palliating existing illness. Throughout the history of public health, preventive measures have been at the core of its work and have constituted the major thrust of its activities. These were first applied to the control of epidemics through community measures such as quarantine and isolation. Later, sanitation measures and immunization followed. The extension of knowledge made possible many methods which are now used as preventive measures in the community.

Health Promotion

Health promotion is disease prevention in the broadest sense, and it is oriented toward behavioral as well as physiological factors. Community health education represents a major effort in this area. Social measures such as those which attempt to provide adequate income, housing, and recreation facilities, healthy working conditions, and adequate nutrition also contribute significantly to disease prevention. Laws, such as those directed at the drunken driver and pollution of the environment, as well as the range of legislation affecting product safety and consumer protection, contribute substantially to protecting the health of the public.

Scope of Public Health

While the focus on prevention continues to be a primary characteristic of public health, two important changes have occurred. One is the application of preventive objectives to a far broader array of health and related social problems than has been the customary responsibility of public health departments. The other is the enlargement of the concept of prevention to include the prevention of the progression of disease in addition to caring for the individual whose private means are not adequate to procure needed care. What is implied by this briefly stated inventory is that the nature of these problems requires solutions that call for actions and organizations well beyond the traditional models of public health department, voluntary organizations, and private initiative and responsibility.

A statement of the elements in contemporary American society that lie within the purview of public health will further specify the Commission's frame of reference. The traditional areas of sanitation and preventive medicine continue to be central. Medical care is now considered to be a component of public health. The physical and social environment of human beings, as a source of hazards or as a potentially positive factor in growth and development, must also be considered a part of public health. This view of the scope and content of public health obviously outruns definitions based on traditional models of disease, organizational roles and responsibilities, or public and private sector concerns.

To say that the boundaries have been extended is not to say that they have disappeared. The sanctions for public health roles and methods ultimately depend on community values. Four important limitations arising from those values in the United States are:

1. The protection of personal liberties and personal dignity as continuously defined and redefined by legislatures and courts.

2. The balance of economic and social benefits and their costs.

3. Existing social assignments of professional responsibility.

4. The nature of the public commitment to social equity.

The Commission is aware that community values are continually changing and that legal definitions are continuously defined and redefined by legislatures and courts. The sanctions for public health activity will also change as these four limitations are further restricted or overcome.

Without assuming overwhelming burdens and infringing inappropriately on the designated responsibilities of other agencies, leaders in public health must ensure that society understands the role which major elements of the standard of living (nutrition, education, housing, employment, etc.) play in determining health status. For example, while public health agencies are not obliged to ensure that each person who so desires is appropriately employed, it is their responsibility to ensure that society understands the role gainful employment plays in promoting and protecting health. In the broadest sense, public health is legitimately concerned with the quality of life, particularly as it manifests itself in the limitation of any individual—because of impaired health status—to maintain his productivity, standard of living, and economic condition.

Public Health Configuration

Public health, therefore, is not a single scientific field organized in a uniform way. It is, rather, a configuration of objectives, policies, resources, and activities that is socially determined by a community, state, or nation. The nature of the organization and programs is pluralistic, and the knowledge base from which it functions is complex, multidisciplinary, and interacting. As this knowledge base continues to broaden, the number of skills and professions pertinent to public health increases, from the beginnings, which were based solely on engineering and medicine, to the present involvement of biomedical sciences, management sciences, social sciences, and the law, among others. Increasingly crucial to the entire public health configuration are special programs of higher education which must be designed to prepare personnel of appropriate professional and technical capacity to function in the increasingly complicated network necessary to achieve the goals of public health.

2. Meeting Health Needs

Higher education for public health is a relatively recent development in the United States. The first school dedicated to this purpose was established in 1916 as the Institute of Hygiene at Johns Hopkins University. At that time, the over-riding public health concerns of the nation centered around the communicable diseases, and education was designed to further their control.

Since then there have been great changes in the nature and scope of health problems. Communicable diseases are no longer a major cause of death in this country, and relatively few young Americans die of diphtheria, measles, tuberculosis, or typhoid fever. While the time-honored methods for controlling these diseases must be maintained, to prevent a recurrence of plagues, public health education and emphases must alter drastically to meet the needs of the immediate future and of the decades to come.

Mortality Rates

The salient feature of national mortality statistics in the twentieth century has been the large decline in deaths during infancy and early childhood, resulting in an increase in life expectancy from 47 years in 1900 to 70 years by 1950 (U.S. Bureau of the Census, 1973; National Center for Health Statistics, 1969). Much of this reduction in mortality took place between 1900 and 1930, with some improvement over the next two decades. Relatively little progress has been made in lowering the death rate since 1950. In spite of overwhelming technologic developments in medicine, the expansion of medical services, and increases in health insurance programs, overall mortality rates have remained virtually stationary since 1960.

Most of the reduction in mortality has been realized through the control of acute and communicable diseases. Traditional public health measures, such as sanitation and mass immunization, later combined with therapeutic breakthroughs in medical care to produce startling triumphs. Improvements in nutrition, housing, and other elements in the general standard of living have undoubtedly had a significant effect.

While national mortality information is useful to identify general trends, it also conceals important differences between groups in the population. At the grossest level, there are significant differences in life expectancy between men and women and between white and nonwhite Americans, with nonwhite males having the shortest life expectancy. In 1969, for example, life expectancy for the United States population as a whole was 70 years (U.S. Bureau of the Census, 1973). White Americans, however, had a life expectancy of 71 years, while for nonwhites the figure was 64 years. Important variations are also to be found according to socioeconomic status and geographic locale, and reflect not only certain possible genetic differences but, more importantly, inadequate implementation of current knowledge. Our society often awards top priority to rugged individualism and to industrial progress, and has only begun to accept a commitment to social equity for racial and other ethnic minorities. Limited sanctions for public health activities are thus often manifest in gross differences between the health of groups.

Causes of death have also changed in their relative importance during the twentieth century. In 1900 pneumonia, tuberculosis, and gastrointestinal diseases were major causes of death, and the childhood infectious diseases, such as measles, diphtheria, and whooping cough, accounted for more deaths than did all cancers (Grove and Hetzel, 1968). These major killers of the past have ceased to be significant threats and three chronic diseases, heart disease, stroke, and cancer, which occur primarily among older people, are now the leading causes of death. These diseases also produce a great deal of disability in the United States today.

There are other diseases and conditions, such as chronic mental diseases, arthritis, and rheumatism which produce large amounts of disability and restricted activity with little mortality. The failure to prevent and effectively treat chronic diseases is largely the result of

lack of precise knowledge concerning their etiology, and of the
multiple contributing factors which affect their patterns of occurrence.

Importance of
the Physical Environment

That the physical environment has an important effect on health
has long been known. Until recently, however, so-called "natural"
variations of occurrences were the primary concern of public health.
Epidemics resulting from the transmission of infectious disease by
food, water, air, and small insects and animals have been controlled,
largely through the efforts of public health and public works agencies
using measures such as water sanitation, solid waste disposal, and
vector control.

Today, public health confronts the effects of man-made hazards,
which have been introduced into the environment largely as by-
products of an explosive technology. Although the extent of the
relationship of these hazards to human health is still not entirely
known, it appears that man-made hazards in the environment may
be increasing at a rate which threatens previous gains in protecting
health and reducing mortality. Their consequences are demonstrated
in three general areas: the production of specific diseases, their
effect on the quality of human life, and their long-term impact
on the ecology of this planet.

Many industrial metals, such as lead, mercury, and manganese,
are cumulative poisons. Exposure of workers to widely used industrial chemicals causes specific diseases, such as bladder cancer
in workers in the aniline dye industry, "black lung" in coal miners,
and liver cancer in vinyl chloride workers. Most often these diseases
affect workers in a particular industry, but asbestos, for example,
affects not only employees of the asbestos factory but also people
who live in the neighborhood of the factory. The presence of
asbestos fibers—a byproduct of refining ore containing taconite—
has been demonstrated in high concentrations in Lake Superior,
and no fewer than 66 chemicals, many of them carcinogenic, have

been found by the Environmental Protection Agency in the water of the Mississippi which is used for drinking by many communities (New York Times, 1974).

Industrial development also affects human health indirectly by influencing the quality of life and the standard of living. Heat, noise, and polluted air directly affect mental and physical well-being. Accidents, the fourth leading cause of death, have been increasing not only because of the greater use of automobiles but also because of the creation and use in industry and at home of new, hazardous products (Hanlon, 1972; Chanlett, 1973).

Another hazard involves the effect of technology on plant and animal life, and on natural resources. A few examples will suffice, such as the potential of discharges from combustion or spray-cans to reduce the layer of ozone in the atmosphere. Measures taken to prevent breeding of the malaria mosquito have resulted in increased populations of other insects, and certain common houseflies have undergone genetic mutation which allows them to tolerate DDT. The effect of DDT on the eggshells of birds is well known, and its extensive use is beginning to cause changes in ecologic balances. The changes in ecology produced by man-made agents will have reciprocal effects on man's health.

It must be emphasized in all discussions of man-made hazards in the environment that the consequences are only partially understood. It is easy to speak of direct relationships and to identify hazards when effects are manifested in a relatively brief time. However, some of the newer chemical and physical agents may exhibit their effects only on future generations in the form of harmful genetic mutation or congenital defects. The dangers of ionizing radiation are well-known in this context.

Over the past 10 years four major commissions have confirmed that the environment in many regions of the United States is deteriorating (Committee on Environmental Health Problems, 1962; President's Science Advisory Committee, Environmental Pollution Panel, 1965; Committee, National Academy of Science, 1966; Task Force on Environmental Health-Related Problems, 1967). Many of the recommendations of these commissions have direct implications for public health professionals. In order to protect and maintain the health of the public, it is imperative to apply present knowledge fully and effectively through societal mechanisms.

Ways of Meeting Health Problems

This summary of the major health problems in the United States today—inequalities in health status, chronic diseases, and environmental hazards—has been necessarily brief and is intended only to serve as an introduction to our discussion of the part public health must play in modern times. Our nation has developed a network of activities to prevent and treat disease and to protect the health of the population, and each aspect of this network has interfaces with public health. It is possible to classify these and discuss them under three general headings: personal medical care, environmental controls, and health promotion or education. Public health organizations and personnel have an important role to play in each of these, and it is expected that our explication of these roles will point to the necessary direction of higher education for public health.

Personal Medical Care

This nation's system for delivery of personal medical care services has been described elsewhere in terms of the numbers of people involved, the substantial investments which have been made, and its often dramatic achievements, and it is unnecessary to give a complete recapitulation here. Certain striking characteristics, however, are worthy of mention.

In contrast to the fairly recent past, when almost all primary care was provided by a family doctor, today a wide range of occupational groups (physicians, nurses, dentists, pharmacists, medical technicians, and other health workers) are engaged in the direct provision of services. New types of manpower, such as nurse practitioners and physician's assistants, are rapidly being added.

Institutional involvement in medical care is also growing. There are now more than 7,000 hospitals (American Hospital Association, 1974) and 16,000 nursing homes (National Center for Health Statistics, 1973a and 1974a) for acute, chronic, and custodial care, and approximately 2,500 certified home health agency outreach programs (National Center for Health Statistics, 1974b) which bring services to patients in their homes.

The financing mechanisms for medical care services have become almost equally diverse and complicated. They include individual payment for services, federal and state programs of Medicare and Medicaid, private medical and hospital insurance systems, and some arrangements for the direct provision of medical services to special groups.

Defects of accessibility, quality, and cost exist in this medical care system, and public health agencies and organizations have key roles to play in their identification and resolution.

Americans do not have equal access to medical care. Financial constraints are an obvious limitation. Maldistribution of medical personnel has produced a deficiency or absence of physicians in many inner city and rural areas, making care unavailable to many people. This maldistribution is compounded by the trend towards specialization, which further limits the accessibility of the physician.

There is a great need for public health leadership to overcome the fragmentation of current distribution systems, to involve the newer health services personnel, and to plan for the allocation of medical resources so that care will be accessible to all who need it

Variations in the quality of medical care services in the United States also exist, ranging from unacceptable or dangerous to adequate or excellent. No assurance of quality can be given without some form of regulation, and in many situations where health and safety are involved, regulatory powers are vested in official public health agencies. At present, however, regulation in the medical care system is fragmented, limited in scope, and usually controlled by professional organizations. Where official agencies are authorized to control licensure and set institutional standards, inspection and enforcement vary in quality and effectiveness.

Professional Standards Review Organizations have recently been mandated to establish criteria for professionally recognized standards for the quality of medical care paid for by federal funds. It is too early to say how much influence these standards will have on care not paid for by the federal government, or how vigorously the PSROs will pursue investigation of apparent substandard practices and practitioners, but certainly their success will depend upon the ability of personnel to evaluate and monitor medical care services.

The cost of health care has become the single most visible health issue to the public. It is clear that the total has been rising rapidly and continues to rise so that today more than 8 percent of the nation's Gross National Product is spent on health care. The burden of costs falls unevenly on different groups of the population, who also differ in their ability to meet such costs. Those groups with the greatest need for services—the chronically ill, the aged, the poor, and those in rural areas—have less insurance coverage and are less able to pay out-of-pocket costs than many who require less medical care. There are also many indications that the benefits obtained are not equal to the costs, and that money is allocated for medical services in response to fortuitous pressures rather than as a result of rational decisions made on the basis of a community perspective.

Federal legislation attempting to fill some of these gaps was passed by Congress in 1965. However, on a nationwide basis the federal Medicare program for persons over the age of 65 currently pays for only 40 percent of the total medical expenditures of the elderly. Medicaid funds to help pay for services to the indigent must be matched, at variable rates, by state and/or local funds, and resulting programs are uneven in the scope of services paid for as well as in the definition of eligibility. For an excellent exposition of this, see Karen Davis (1975).

The federal government is also engaged in the direct provision of comprehensive services for selected groups: members of the armed forces, veterans, and American Indians—14 million Americans. Some states and municipalities also provide some programs of direct medical care, usually to income- or disease-related categories.

In spite of these programs, there are strong indications that only national health insurance can remove the economic barrier which prevents many people from obtaining the care they need. National debate centers not only on the methods of financing, the locus of administration, and the scope of services to be covered, but also on whether the plan should take responsibility for the organization of services so that these will be optimally effective and economic. How this debate is resolved will determine whether national health insurance will be only a financing mechanism or a lever for the development of a more comprehensive and integrated national health policy.

Whatever decisions are made about financing methods, quality controls, and equalizing access to medical care services, there is no doubt that the tendency for personal medical services to be delivered through some form of organized system is increasing. Whether these systems are public or private does not affect the need for people who will be able to monitor quality of care, set rational funding policies, and function in planning, evaluative, and administrative capacities. This will intensify the existing need for public health personnel, as no matter what system is instituted, policy decisions will have to be made and implemented, and skilled professional planners, managers, and administrators will be essential.

Environmental Controls

The scope of activity concerning the environment has greatly increased in the past two decades, and a series of new agencies has been set up to deal with the many things in our environment, both natural and man-made, which may be hazardous to human health.

A variety of enabling legislation has been enacted as part of this nation's effort to preserve the quality of the environment. The Environmental Policy Act of 1969 makes environmental protection a matter of national policy, and sets out our environmental objectives on an international basis in cooperation with other nations. Specific health-related environmental legislation includes the Air Quality Act, the Water Pollution Control Act, the Solid Waste Disposal Act, the Environmental Pesticide Control Act, and the Noise Control Act. The Occupational Safety and Health Act of 1970 covers more than four million workplaces in the nation and authorizes enforcement of standards set under the Act to ensure safe and healthy working conditions for men and women.

In the past, responsibility for controlling the harmful effects of the environment on the health of people rested chiefly with state and local health departments, which were charged with ensuring pure water and food supplies, the control of noxious substances in the air, and safe waste and sewage disposal. Although activities and knowledge were more limited than they are today, this arrangement meant that public health professionals made most of the decisions about needed actions concerning the environment, and that available information about health effects was central to these decisions.

Today many different kinds of agencies are concerned with the environment. On the national level, the Environmental Protection Agency is involved primarily with programs designed to abate pollution and protect the overall environment. On the state level, 29 states have placed the general environmental protection function in some department other than the department of health. These agencies and departments have a variety of titles, such as Department of Environmental Protection (Connecticut, Illinois, Maine, New Jersey), Department of Air and Water Pollution Control (Florida), Department of Resources and Recreation (Wyoming), and Pollution Control Agency (Minnesota) (personal communications with, and data transmitted by, Mr. Paul Hibbard).

At the local level, environmental control activities are still largely the responsibility of health departments, although many large cities have established separate agencies to deal with special problems such as air pollution or noise control. There are also several regional agencies which have been set up to cope with some of the many environmental factors which are not contained by, or within, political boundary lines. The Tri-State Transportation Commission, for example, is responsible for problems of solid waste in three states (New York, New Jersey, and Connecticut). The Delaware River Basin Commission is concerned with the water supply problems of four states (Delaware, Pennsylvania, New York, and New Jersey).

There are some sound reasons for removing environmental problems from the sole aegis of the health department and placing them in the context of a broader or specialized and distinct authority. With the increased development of technology and greater industrialization and urbanization of our nation, control of the environment is closely involved with questions of economic interests. There is a growing number of pollutants produced by the synthesis of chemical elements into new products, and the concentration of population in large cities has made more people vulnerable to resulting potential hazards from industrial pollution. The nature of environmental control has changed from the relatively simple matter of purifying a water supply to prevent disease, to larger and more complex problems which involve making sure that there is any water supply at all for many communities. However, this expansion of the area of environmental concern does not reduce the need for adequate consideration of health factors pertinent to the solution of problems. There is still a great need for public health representation in all activities for control of the environment, to make sure that proper attention is given to the health effects of hazards and the adoption of measures to eliminate them.

Environmental control involves many technicians and professional people in a range of activities. It is estimated that more than 243,000 people are employed in environmental health activities. These include environmental engineers, who may specialize in areas such as air pollution control, industrial hygiene, radiation and hazard control, and sanitary engineering, and sanitarians who perform a wide range of duties including inspection of food manufacturing and processing plants, dairies, and water supplies. There is also a number of environmental health program specialists, such as industrial hygiene and radiation protection personnel, while chemists, toxicologists, physicists, and biologists may work with non-professional personnel as members of environmental protection teams (National Center for Health Statistics, 1973b).

The activities aimed at ensuring a safe and pleasant environment are substantial and increasing. There is cause for concern, however, that the quality of the environment may be deteriorating faster than control measures can compensate. Science, industry, and government tend to view each environmental hazard separately. This ignores the fact that human beings are not exposed to one substance alone but to a spectrum of cumulative hazards, each of which might be minimal, but the total burden of which might be critical or overwhelming.

Environmental problems have two aspects, the scientific on the one hand, and the economic and sociopolitical on the other. The latter are likely to be the most intractable. For example, if pollution control in an industry makes plant operations unprofitable and thus results in a loss of jobs, the ensuing unemployment, financial distress, and possible impaired nutrition of workers' families might be more detrimental to health and well-being than the original pollution. In the future the public will be called upon with increasing frequency to make decisions of the utmost gravity which will involve balancing health gains against the economic and sociopolitical costs of meeting them. There are no easy answers to the questions that must be faced. The need for the full involvement of appropriate public health expertise is clearly essential.

Health Promotion and Education

Programs to improve the health of populations cannot rely solely on the activities of health professionals and the health services delivery system. People must take individual action to protect and improve their health, and to prevent disability and premature death.

The major health problems today are those of chronic disease and environmentally-related illness. The control of these not uncommonly involves long-term changes in living habits or in the economic and cultural fabric of the nation. Individual initiative and behavioral change are necessary ingredients of prevention, treatment, and rehabilitation.

The control of chronic illness requires a new approach to medical care by the health professions, and a new kind of responsibility for preventive behavior by the population. The best long-term solution to chronic personal health problems is dependent on prevention, and on the containment and reduction of disability. Such services are not yet well integrated with medical care practice. In addition, the successful management of chronic conditions is often dependent upon adherence to a prescribed diet, long-term complex drug therapy, or a specified regimen for daily activity. These measures call for a radical change in the patient's pattern of living, and involve the breaking of ingrained habits which contribute to the continuation of the chronic condition. Consequently, the prevention and treatment of chronic disease require behavioral change on the part of individuals. Such a change is often the major factor determining the prognosis and final outcome of the chronic disease process.

In the case of accidents, as with certain chronic diseases, prevention may perhaps be more effectively accomplished through manipulation of the physical and social environment than through attempts to change behavior. For example, in the winter of 1974 the nation experienced a "natural experiment" in environmental change through the lowering of the automobile speed limits to 55 mph. This change, plus reduced amounts of travel, lowered the death toll from automobile accidents for 1974 by 20 percent, a saving of 11,000 lives in that year (communications from the National Safety Council, 1975). Hopes for reversing the upward trend in the death rate from chronic obstructive pulmonary disease (now the tenth leading cause of death) may lie with reducing exposure to inhaled pollutants, whether by industrial and other controls, or by a reduction in cigarette smoking. These observations involve us with problems of policy and value judgments, where the choices are not made by health professionals alone.

Equally important is the fact that community, state, and national action cannot be taken without public understanding and support. When people understand the valid reasons for a procedure or program they can be mobilized to support it. There are many examples where this has happened, ranging from the early conflicts over the chlorination of public water supplies to the more recent disagreements about fluoridation. Although some segments of the public were initially frightened by the idea of adding chemicals to drinking water, educational efforts succeeded in changing their attitudes, and today chlorination is an accepted procedure which contributes significantly to the health of our population. Fluoridation, too, is gradually being accepted in many parts of the nation.

Efforts to educate the public about health are now being made by many different agencies in the United States. Public health departments at all levels use education to attempt to generate an understanding of new problems, to provide support for new programs, to induce people to utilize services after they have been instituted, and also to produce a better understanding on the part of the public of certain diseases in which individual understanding and cooperation are crucial. Voluntary organizations concerned with the prevention and treatment of a particular disease produce a mass of educational material in their areas of special interest. Many hospitals have developed materials which explain hospital procedures so that patients will be informed about their hospital stay. Professional associations and others have made substantial efforts to provide instructional materials, particularly in the area of diet and regimen, for doctors to use in their education of patients about diseases and therapy.

Health educators are public health professionals who promote the health of the public through education. They plan or direct educational programs for other health personnel, develop educational strategies and, as members of health agencies, analyze sociological, cultural, and situational factors affecting behavioral changes needed for the solution of health problems. They function in community organization, dissemination of information, and the further education of a wide variety of health professionals. They also organize and administer the educational aspects of health programs.

Most health education programs are aimed at specific diseases. Few of them attempt to produce public understanding of basic health issues. However, evidence suggests that the public is more ready to accept innovation in the health care system than is generally assumed, and even more ready than the health professional. The public is now demanding a greater share of the responsibility for determining the quality of its own health care. The consumer movement, for example, appears to stem from personal and social motivation to control and participate in the health care system in a role other than that of the sick patient. People of all socioeconomic levels want greater involvement in planning for facilities, programs, delivery of services and the development of priorities in the health system.

In the past, public health professionals were able to exert substantial influence on community health standards by working through federal regulatory agencies, local government, and nongovernmental organizations, voluntary societies and self-help groups. Partly as a result of their efforts, state and the federal government set policies in such areas as institutional licensing, sewage treatment, radiation and noise levels, and immunization programs for school-aged children. These programs could be implemented by health professionals and were based upon firm scientific knowledge. Once the public was informed and convinced of the beneficial effects of a recommended procedure such as the chlorination of water supplies, public health professionals were empowered to organize and carry out a program to achieve the desired benefits.

It has been suggested that professional influence on, and control of, the nature of health programs is lessening, as health care and health education decisions are more and more frequently politicized. The importance of the political arena must be recognized, and health educators must be prepared to work with decision makers or to help others who must influence decision makers. Where in the past health educators, like most other public health professionals, may have avoided overt engagement in the politics of delivery of health care services, they can no longer afford to maintain this position. Indeed, if health decisions are being made in the political arena, all health professionals must seek active involvement with the public in the formation of political solutions.

3. Public Health Activities
and Organizations

It is clear that public health is an integral part of all three kinds of efforts now used to meet our nation's health problems: the personal medical care system, the environmental control network, and health promotion and health education. Recognition of this has led to an expansion of public health activities which began at the turn of the century and has accelerated during the past 25 years. The expansion began almost as soon as a pressing need for health departments was generally recognized.

Examples of the kinds of activities now carried out, but not visualized in early concepts of public health functions, can be derived from a review of some recent federal legislation. In 1965 Congress established programs providing for health insurance for the aged, and an expanded and unified program of grants to states for medical assistance for the indigent. Also in 1965 the Regional Medical Programs established grants to plan and develop regional cooperative arrangements by public and nonprofit groups for demonstration, training, and research in patient care in the fields of heart disease, cancer, stroke, and related diseases. In 1966 the Comprehensive Health Planning and Services Act introduced the concept of comprehensive health planning as a mechanism through which the planning activities of all those concerned with health services could be linked. The National Health Planning and Resources Development Act of 1974 altered and strengthened this mandate. These legislative actions not only legitimize the inclusion of new functions in public health (such as planning for health facilities and resources, the financing and provision of medical care, and direct medical services) but also recognize the important relationships between official and nonofficial agencies and institutions.

As the parameters of public health have expanded, so the organization of public health work has become more diversified. Until the 1960s public health activity was generally thought to be work carried out by the United States Public Health Service, by state and local health departments, and by some voluntary health organizations. The institutional and organizational forms of public health efforts have changed greatly, and in the past decade a plethora of new agencies has appeared (environmental protection agencies, neighborhood health centers, community mental health centers, etc.) which has enriched the fabric of public health and burst the boundaries of traditional health departments. Change in the allocation of responsibility between government and nongovernment agencies continues to take place. Nevertheless, some description of the development and structure of the organizations with a primary responsibility for public health activities seems in order.

Federal Organization for Public Health

For more than a century and a half the United States Public Health Service, headed by the Surgeon General, was the focal point for national public health activities. Established in 1798 as the Marine Hospital Service, it was reorganized in 1912 to coordinate and administer major federal health programs. This more comprehensive Public Health Service was authorized to enforce quarantine laws, to cooperate with states and communities in the control of communicable disease, and to study and regulate the growing problems of urbanization, such as hygiene, sanitation, and water pollution. Federal legislation continued to assign additional health duties to the Public Health Service under the Social Security Act of 1935, which systematized assistance to the states for health manpower development, disease control programs, and limited medical care. With the formation of the Department of Health, Education, and Welfare in 1953, this pre-eminent role was diminished and more recent changes have virtually eliminated the Public Health Service, as such.

Drastic reorganizations in the Department of Health, Education, and Welfare have occurred so frequently in recent years that any description of this year's organizational structure may be out of date next year. Nevertheless, by July 1975 it was clear that the Surgeon General no longer functioned as head of the Public Health

Service. Instead, the office of Assistant Secretary for Health of HEW had been strengthened, with six units, formerly the responsibility of the Public Health Service, now accountable to him. These are:

1. National Institutes of Health.
2. Food and Drug Administration.
3. Health Resources Administration.
4. Center for Disease Control.
5. Health Services Administration.
6. Alcohol, Drug Abuse, and Mental Health Administration.

These official health agencies account for only a portion of the health activities of the federal government, which are widely distributed throughout various departments, bureaus and agencies. Virtually every major department of the federal government has responsibility for, and jurisdiction over some type of health activity.

This proliferation within the federal government often leaves Congress, as well as state and local public health workers, confused as to who is responsible for what. Organizational changes continue at a bewildering rate, and involve major decisions about state and local relationships. For many years the Surgeon General of the U.S. Public Health Service and his staff worked directly with state health officers, who in turn worked directly with local health officers. Communication channels were narrow but reasonably effective. As the overriding problems of large cities became more and more urgent, it often became expedient for the federal agency to work directly with cities and other local units, thus bypassing the state health departments. This broadened the channels of communication and increased local community involvement, but it is now often difficult to understand what is happening in large urban areas, where interrelationships with federal agencies are so complex that it often takes much time and energy to unravel the mechanism for providing a service.

State Health Organization

State legislatures define the organizations in each state responsible for health activity. Such laws differ from state to state. In all 50 states there is provision for some type of supervisory Board of Health.

Each state has a state health department or its equivalent to carry out a variety of programs and services, either through direct provision of services or through arrangements with local health units (Association of State and Territorial Health Officials, 1975a). The effort is a sizeable one, and in fiscal 1974 state health agencies expended 2.3 billion dollars for public health programs (The Association of State and Territorial Health Officials, 1975b). Traditional communicable disease programs offer immunization services, venereal disease screening and treatment, and tuberculosis control measures. In addition, there are chronic disease programs of screening, consultation, and treatment, and special programs for alcohol and drug addiction, dental care for children, and services for special groups in the population. Environmental control programs include radiation safety, vector control, water quality, occupational health and safety, and general sanitation. Vital statistics and other kinds of demographic data relating to health are collected, monitored, and analyzed, and relevant information is publicized.

State health agencies are also involved in setting standards for the quality of health care, licensure, and certification of health facilities and manpower, regulating, containing, and reducing costs of health care, and attempts to compensate for the geographic maldistribution of health care providers.

Responsibilities for programs in certain fields are frequently administratively located in different agencies in different states. For example, state mental health programs are located in separate departments of mental health, departments of welfare, departments of human resources, departments of hospitals and institutions, as well as in the state health departments. In more than half the states, many environmental protection functions are now located in departments of environmental protection, natural resources, or pollution control.

Another confusing factor in trying to understand state health organizations is that more than one agency often has responsibility in a given field. More than 60 different types of state agencies contribute in some way to state health programs. Reorganizations occur and new names are given to existing agencies with increasing frequency. Although human resources agencies, environmental protection agencies, and health service agencies represent new organizational responses to public need, in many jurisdictions it is virtually impossible to locate a single agency fully responsible for dealing with a particular health problem.

Local Health Agencies

There are tens of thousands of units of local government in the United States: counties, municipalities, townships, school districts, and special districts. These overlap each other jurisdictionally, and there are vast differences in size and population from one unit to another.

It is possible to say that in 1974 there were more than 2,300 local health departments (Health Services Research Center and School of Public Health of the University of North Carolina at Chapel Hill, and Milbank Memorial Fund Commission, 1974), but it is probably not valid to rank a gigantic municipal department with a large budget, numerous programs, and hundreds of employees in the same category as a tiny department with few resources. However, no matter what the size, the local department has little authority beyond that prescribed by the state.

Three major roles have frequently been described for state and local health departments: planning, regulation and control, and delivery of services. The first two have become, and are likely to remain, state functions, with local departments chiefly responsible for much of their implementation and for the delivery of direct health services.

The local health department serves as the chief consultant and advisor to local government officials and local or regional planning bodies as they consider important health-related decisions. Similarly, local units serve state and federal agencies with responsibilities for health laws, regulations, and/or policy formulation.

The local health departments are responsible for the enforcement of many state laws and regulations, particularly in the environmental health field (i.e., ensuring safe water supply, sewage disposal, and solid waste collection and disposal) and for monitoring standards of sanitation in restaurants, lodging houses, and other institutions. In addition, local health departments serve as official registrars of births and deaths, and keep track of the occurrence of unusual diseases and epidemics.

Local health departments provide direct medical care services for prevention or treatment required by law or mandated by tradition, either by disease category or for specified target populations. Many ambulatory care programs for otherwise unserved sections of the community have been developed under their aegis.

Now that the traditional role of local health departments in the control of communicable disease has been almost universally achieved, many people have begun to question the relevance of such departments. In the last decade or more, many local health departments have been slow to move on new problems, and other voluntary and public agencies have moved into these fields. The failure of health departments to innovate is reflected in the use of other agencies at state and local levels (such as environmental protection agencies, separate agencies for community mental health services, and social welfare departments) to deal with newer issues.

There is, however, an important place for local responsibility and administration of public health services in jurisdictions large enough to support an efficient organization. Even though central financing, and federal and state standards necessarily form the basis of public health programs, most of the activities are carried out at the local community level. To be successful, the understanding, cooperation, and acceptance of the people being served is needed. Therefore, local agencies have a role that cannot be carried out as well from more remote levels.

Voluntary Agencies

Numerous voluntary health agencies and institutions have made a major contribution to the identification of health problems and the development of programs to help solve them. They constitute a major element in the network of health organizations in this nation.

It has been reported that there are more than 100,000 voluntary agencies in the U.S. involved in health and welfare activities. These vary in size and influence from the large national voluntary agencies and foundations to the small local agencies providing a single service in a community, such as the Visiting Nurse Association. Many of these organizations, such as the American Cancer Society and the American Heart Association, began with the sole purpose of fund raising to aid sufferers from a particular disease, and have since expanded their programs to include physician and community health education, research, and program planning. Similar contributions have been made by the National Tuberculosis Association, the American Social Hygiene Association, The National Foundation, and the National Association of Crippled Children and Adults, to name but a few. Such organizations have played, and continue to play, a key role in the development of health programs to meet the public's needs in their fields of interest. They have developed a positive functional interaction with government programs, and demonstrate effective partnerships between the public and the private sector in our society.

Several foundations with a major interest in public health, such as the Rockefeller Foundation, the Commonwealth Fund, the W.K. Kellogg Foundation, and the Milbank Memorial Fund, have played a significant role in developing and promoting the role of health departments, and in supporting basic research in public health and educational programs to prepare professional personnel for this field. These foundations and others like them have modified their goals in public health as the problems have changed.

Voluntary professional associations, supported through membership fees, such as the American Medical Association, the National League for Nursing, the American Hospital Association, and the American Public Health Association took on the responsibility of setting standards for the quality of professional education and performance. Just after World War II, the Joint Commission on the Accreditation of Hospitals, a voluntary coalition of several of these organizations, developed and implemented a national program of hospital accreditation which is now used by government agencies.

Voluntary community hospitals were founded to provide institutional facilities and services for medical care that would otherwise not be available in the community. Though their base is local, they are now considered as part of the larger hospital "system" and are expected to respond to the health needs of the community *qua* community. The increasing proportion of funds that they collect from government and from such quasipublic organizations as Blue Cross, means that increasingly they must be responsive and accountable to a broader constituency than their own boards of trustees. Consumer groups are applying pressure on the issues of quality, access to care, and containment of costs. Here, too, the need to modify and strengthen the interaction and interdependence of the public and the private sectors is emerging sharply.

Organizations such as Blue Cross and Blue Shield, whose original purpose was to make group arrangements for payment for the care given to individuals, have also begun to expand their activities. They are now involved in monitoring the quality of care, preventing unnecessary duplication of resources, and stimulating the development of new forms of service, such as units for ambulatory surgery and organized home care services.

Voluntary agencies and organizations have helped to uncover health needs, to demonstrate and develop solutions, to provide care, to educate the public and the health professions, and to propound legislation and organized efforts to promote the health of the community. All these activities are of a quasipublic nature and they constitute public health activities as defined by the Commission, for they involve organized efforts to protect and restore the health of the public.

Major Issues in the Solution
of Health Problems

Clearly, the health needs of the American people have changed during this century to the point where the institutional responses of earlier decades are inadequate and, in some respects, insensitive to the problems. Traditional public health programs of sanitation and communicable disease control must of course be maintained and strengthened so that the gains of the past are not lost. It is shocking to read of inadequate purification of water supplies in some of our large cities, or of the lack of immunization of many American children. In the light of the demonstrated value of control measures, these shortcomings raise serious questions about the nation's appreciation of public health programs as well as about the effectiveness of the agencies responsible for carrying them out. Recent epidemics of diphtheria or outbreaks of typhoid fever in our cities are inexcusable and simply mean that available preventive and control measures are not being fully applied.

In spite of the sizable effort of the large numbers of agencies, organizations and professional personnel, the role of public health activity is inadequately recognized in our nation today. Awareness of the field of public health usually emerges only when an acute problem, such as an epidemic, threatens. Most public health activities are carried out on a routine basis. When successful, they contain and limit problems. When diseases or environmental hazards are prevented or controlled, it is easy to forget their existence and to ignore the knowledge, skills, and the methods that have achieved this desirable result.

The patterns of illness and mortality in the United States today suggest that personal medical care services alone will not be able to solve all the nation's health problems. This conclusion is based on the realization that, without the necessary changes in social, environmental, and individual living patterns, even the most sophisticated medical care has little effect on the major contributors to mortality. For most chronic diseases, accidents, and the effects of toxic agents and environmental pollution, personal medical care only ameliorates physical damage after the fact. Though we do not yet have the information to deal with these problems completely, some preventive measures and appropriate treatment can be found by changing living patterns and social circumstances and by the effective organization of health services.

Definitive solutions for these problems are neither simple nor always close at hand. But, as a nation, we cannot close our eyes and hope that our major health problems will go away. If we do not apply the knowledge that we now have, and do not approach these issues in a coherent and systematic way, there will be serious consequences in the near future, and the health of the American people will suffer accordingly.

More effective public health programs are essential at every level if progress is to be made. The best approach to overcoming chronic disease today is through prevention, which often requires that individuals must assume responsibility for maintaining their own health. Public action is essential for any real control of environmental hazards. Reorganization of our medical care system on a massive scale is essential if we are to make more health services accessible to more people at reasonable cost.

We recognize that lack of knowledge impairs our ability to deal effectively with many of these issues. Health promotion, and health education of the public, though successful with some of our past major health problems, do not yet produce substantial behavioral change, especially as far as cigarette smoking and dietary practices are concerned. In spite of the many official agencies and new policies that have been developed to control environmental hazards, new pollutants appear to be introduced faster than the old ones can be controlled or eliminated. Certainly, political resistance and conflict over the rationalization of our health services system reflect an absence of some essential tools of implementation and administration.

An adequate supply of professional personnel, appropriately trained to carry out a wide range of technical and professional public health activities, is fundamental to success. The Commission does not believe that technology and managerial skill will, of themselves, solve the health problems of our nation. Health policy issues must first be addressed effectively. But as those issues become more complex, more expertise is needed. In addition to personnel with specialized training in the specific fields that contribute to public health, there is an acute need for people who are trained to cope with the broad concepts of social policy as these affect health. It is essential that a cadre of professional personnel be developed who can:

—assess the health problems of the community as a whole and
establish priorities in health programs;
—identify the modifiable forces which limit the people's health;

—appraise the means available to foster, protect, and restore health and so delineate precise health goals;

—assemble and organize resources into programs to achieve those goals;

—evaluate progress and develop appropriate modifications.

Pressing national health needs call for responsive change in the system of higher education for public health. Trained people by themselves will not be able to solve all the problems we are now faced with. But without them, the disorder and fragmentation we see today will be even worse tomorrow, and this is something the nation cannot afford.

Recommendation

1. A concerted national effort should be undertaken to develop a larger and better qualified cadre of professional personnel capable of coping with the complex and changing health problems of the nation. Because higher education for public health is a national concern, the responsibility for this endeavor should be shared by federal and state governments, educational institutions, and operating health agencies.

II: Education
for Public Health

4. Personnel
for Public Health

As public health organizations and activities have multiplied and become more complex, the kinds of personnel and skills needed to carry out public health work have increased not only in numbers but also in diversity.

The Physician-Health Officer

Seventy-five years ago it was axiomatic that the key figure in public health was, and always would be, the health officer, and ideally that health officer would be a physician. Although the position of the medically qualified public health practitioner is still pre-eminent, the field has become characterized by greater collegiality. A review of the composition of the membership of the American Public Health Association is indirectly indicative of these changes. In 1898, for example, 80 percent of the 568 members were physicians. By 1968, although the number of physician members had increased to 6,380, they represented only 29 percent of the membership (Terris, 1973). Similarly, 61 percent of all students admitted to schools of public health for the Master of Public Health degree in 1946–47 were physicians, but by 1968–69 physicians constituted only 19 percent of these candidates (Hall et al., 1973a). This is a result of the increase in the scope of public health activities, the variety of organizations engaged in public health work, and the development and employment of an ever-broadening range of specialized professions and technologies.

In the early years of this century, the physician-health officer functioned as a general practitioner in public health. Since then, specialization in public health has followed in the footsteps of clinical medicine, and parasitologists are no more interchangeable with medical care administrators than are brain surgeons with dermatologists. Specialization has affected the entire range of personnel involved in public health. Historically, the physician-health officer with a large enough constituency would be assisted by a sanitarian. Today there are environmental engineers in public health, as well as environmental technologists, sanitarians, and industrial hygienists, each of whom is trained in a highly specialized technique or field of knowledge.

Professional Categories

Three major categories—administrators, nurses, and physicians—account for more than half the positions of people in public health (personal communications with Mr. Harold Cary). These titles, however, fail to describe adequately the range and overlap of activities actually performed by an individual in that category.

The director of the Bureau of Maternal and Child Health in a large urban health department, for example, will most probably be a physician who will function as chief executive of a sizable organization, responsible for many different clinical and research activities, and for developing programs and policies to be carried out by different kinds of staff members and specialists. The physician who examines babies in a well-baby clinic, however, has purely clinical responsibilities. Both are "physicians," but that professional title alone does not illuminate either the character of their work or the educational preparation each needs to operate effectively. Both need adequate knowledge of pediatrics, but the clinician needs relatively less public health orientation than the director of Maternal and Child Health who must be educated to function in a wide range of occupational roles and organizational settings in public health.

Many different disciplines and professions contribute to public health activities. These include medicine, nursing, dentisty, veterinary medicine, engineering, law, social work, and other physical and social sciences. People trained in one of these disciplines, however, will not always function the same way in public health. While some provide the usual services of their particular specialty to a public health program, others will use their profession as a point of departure for broader public health responsibilities. Thus, the professional base and title alone do not adequately convey the nature of the public health task.

Education Determined by Function

The Commission's definition of public health emphasizes those activities mandated, and deliberately organized, by society to protect, promote, and restore the health and quality of life of the people. We have addressed ourselves to the educational needs of personnel who function in ways that are specific to the achievement of these aims. It is the nature of the personnel's tasks, rather than the goal orientation of the organization employing the personnel, which determines the need for education for public health. Thus, not all those who work in a public health setting should be considered public health workers. For example, technical and clerical personnel employed in a public health setting function as they would in any other employment setting. In contrast, the physician who is an expert in occupational medicine and who actively promotes health and safety programs should be considered a public health professional even though these activities are incidental to the major goals of the industrial employer.

This may raise the question of whether or not the director of an institution, such as a hospital or nursing home, is a public health worker. Increasingly, in recent years, hospitals are being considered by the public and the government as having a public health function, in that they are expected to be directly responsive to community-wide needs. It is therefore desirable that administrators of these institutions should have the orientation and training to enable them to function in this different and broader role.

Education for public health must be directed to the task, and not conceived of as related solely to professional categories. The

Commission finds that in all public health programs three kinds of functions can be identified:

1. *Supportive functions*: provided by clerical staff, paraprofessionals, or persons with bachelor's degrees in the arts and sciences. Workers at this level do not need special higher education for public health.

2. *Professional functions*: there are two kinds of professional functions.

(*a*) The first uses people from many different disciplines, such as medicine, nursing, dentistry, social work, law, and engineering, who apply the knowledge and skills of their profession directly or with some slight adaptation, to the field of public health. Some orientation to public health may be part of the basic preparation in each of their disciplines, but is not essential in order for them to fulfill their respective functions in public health.

(*b*) The second uses professionals whose knowledge and skills are centered primarily on public health problems and programs, such as biostatisticians, epidemiologists, public health nurses, nutritionists, health educators, health administrators, and environmental specialists. Higher education for public health is a basic and essential component of their preparation; the scope and depth of such education will vary with the individual specialty and the level of responsibility at which the individual will be functioning.

3. *Executive functions*: these management functions are assumed by executives, policy makers, and planners, all of whom should have broad expertise in the field of public health generally, or in one of the specialties of public health practice. These leaders will probably have training in any one of a number of fields before entering public health. Though such leaders arrive at their positions by a variety of pathways, substantial advanced education for public health is crucial to the success of their future performance.

The Commission has found that this schematization, while relatively simple and straightforward, contains some semantic traps. Can't an "executive" be a "professional?" Doesn't a health administrator in the "professional" category also belong in the "executive" category? Doesn't the administrator plan, formulate, and perform management functions? The answer to these questions, of course, is "Yes." But the knowledge and skills needed to administer an established organization on a day-to-day basis are not the same as those required of leaders who have to review, modify, and develop the appropriate resources to deal with the health problems of a community. Many people use the terms "management" and "administration" interchangeably. Both refer to a basic organizational process which in essence deals with a planned approach to solving problems, and involves a series of functions such as planning, directing, coordinating, and evaluating. Public administration as a discipline/vocation/perspective has tended to use the term "administration" to describe this basic process—while business administration as a discipline/vocation/perspective uses the term "management."

Unfortunately both terms fail to differentiate between various tasks that need to be performed at different levels of organization. This report uses the term "management" to refer to top echelon executive and leadership activities where the primary focus is the relationship of the organization vis-à-vis its environment and the internal integration of various components of the organization itself (Katz and Kahn, 1966). The emphasis at this level is on developing policy, setting priorities, allocating resources, and modifying and manipulating organizational structure. "Administration", for the purposes of this report, refers to ongoing activities at lower levels of organization. Here the focus is on maximizing the existing structure and resources for efficient operation, to accomplish the designated goals of the organization.

The director of a state or local health department, the director of a chronic disease or maternal and child health program in a state or region, and the executive director of a health planning agency can be considered managers in the level, scope, and range of their responsibilities and activities. The director of a small community hospital or long-term care facility, the director of a health maintenance organization, and the director of a local drug addiction program are all administrators whose major responsibilities are carried out in defined and limited institutional settings.

Executive functions also derive, in part, from the size and complexity of the organization. A professional who functions as a specialist in a small agency—as sanitarian or environmental engineer, for example—will probably need new and expanded knowledge and skills to perform adequately in a larger setting. In addition to increased staff and more complicated relationships with others in the community, a broader view of environmental problems needs to be taken than would be required in a smaller setting. The leader of an environmental health team must be capable of integrating the contributions of biomedical researchers, environmental scientists, engineers, and community leaders, and of organizing and directing the efforts of a team composed of various disciplines, all aimed at estimating the nature and magnitude of the public health risk associated with alternative technologies. The depth and breadth of the training and experience required of these leaders for the development and implementation of effective programs are largely determined by the complexity and growing importance of these issues.

The public health leaders who perform managerial functions in any specialty must be able to:

1. *Identify health-related problems in the community*, which involves the quantification and evaluation of data relating to health trends within populations.

2. *Develop and set health priorities*, both for their own organizations and for the community at large.

3. *Formulate policy and make decisions* as well as provide judgemental input into the formulation of social policy for the health arena.

4. *Perform management and administrative functions* in order to organize, administer, and review the effectiveness of those agencies and activities for which they are responsible.

5. *Educate the community* to recognize, and cooperate in serving, its health needs. The public health official is responsible for bringing health concerns to the attention not only of the public at large, but to professional and governmental bodies as well.

6. *Advise and consult and support* community service programs by providing them with information and guidance on the health

aspects of their activities, and by assimilating and coordinating information received from nonpublic health sources.

7. *Perform research and/or evaluate activities* in public health, and encourage the development of new knowledge in fields affecting the health of populations.

Thus, the Commission finds that the many different skills and professions needed in public health can be differentiated into two types of manpower to which the educational system must address itself. The first comprises the large group of people who will be experts at what they do, but who perform within the confines of set priorities and allocated resources; the second group, the leadership cadre, is necessarily smaller, and must establish the framework within which the first group operates, by setting goals and determining policies.

We realize that we are, in fact, dealing with a continuum of people who move from one level of responsibility to another because of opportunity or talent. However, we believe it is valuable to give attention in the plan of the educational program, to the substantial differences in range, scope, and nature of the responsibilities of management and administration.

It is both impossible and unnecessary to provide all elements of the knowledge base equally to all who will work in public health. Different mixes are appropriate for different people, depending upon the responsibilities they will have. The Commission finds that those who will function as policy makers, managers, planners, or educators must acquire the broadest education for public health, as their activities will require an understanding of the entire field. Those who will function in specialty capacities will need varying amounts of education in their defined area, and less in the broader foundation for policy making in public health.

Manpower Needs

It is the Commission's judgment, supported by available data, that the demand for public health manpower will continue to outweigh the supply to such an extent that the current levels of production are, at the least, necessary and desirable.[1] After reviewing a series of reports on utilization and need for public health manpower, we found the most useful compilation and synthesis for our purposes to be that prepared under the direction of Dr. Thomas L. Hall at the University of North Carolina at Chapel Hill. These manpower projections were developed as part of testimony requested by the House of Representatives Subcommittee on Public Health and the Environment on July 24, 1973, and were published as a report entitled *Professional Health Manpower for Community Health Programs 1973* (Hall et al., 1973a). In this document, the projections were claimed to be conservative and to avoid unrealistic assumptions or standards. Only limited public health manpower categories were considered, and the projections assumed continuing federal support which would permit graduate education at roughly the same levels as during the early 1970s. These projections were presented as rough dimensions of need, and not as target figures. The Commission did not undertake a detailed study of its own because of the magnitude and complexity of such an endeavor and the limited time available.

The Commission believes that the changing nature of the health services delivery system will increase the need for individuals who are able to address themselves to public and community, rather than to individual, health problems. Federal policy with regard to the health delivery system is moving toward more administrative decentralization, increased use of allied health manpower, strengthened program management and evaluation, and greater availability of comprehensive health services through new insurance mechanisms. All of these are likely to increase the demand for individuals with preparation in public health. The magnitude of the projected gap in every public health category is so large that there appears to

[1] As a basis for discussing national manpower needs, the Commission reviewed the several studies providing quantitative projections of need for the various professional disciplines active in public health, and data on numbers and employment. Caveats accompanying the statistics on present employment of public health personnel (problems of definition, disparate methodology, inadequate historical documentation) often reduced the validity of the data, making projections speculative.

be little danger of a surplus of public health personnel in the next decade.

Recent federal legislation calling for specified planning activities at federal, state, and local levels (the National Health Planning and Resources Development Act of 1974, for example), or the promotion of Health Maintenance Organizations, and implementation of the Professional Standards Review requirements, will all increase the demand for public health manpower. Certainly there will be, sooner or later, legislation extending health insurance to all citizens. The problems of chronic care services, institutional and home care, will not be neglected too much longer, and will also call for specially qualified manpower. In areas such as occupational safety and environmental controls, the increased need for manpower is already felt. It may be that some new programs will increase the requirements for professional public health specialists in one area and decrease them in another, but on balance we believe there will be a rapid increase in the already growing demand for health care professionals at all levels.

Projections in Selected Health Manpower Categories

The Commission critically reviewed the 1980 projections (Table 1) in the 1973 report cited above. In spite of the risks of making estimates in this field, the Commission believes that the logic underlying these approximations is sound, and the projections provide a guide for the foreseeable future. The report prepared under Dr. Hall's direction utilized secondary source data and statistics exclusively. Current employment figures and projected requirements/deficits of health professionals were based upon data garnered from government agencies, private and voluntary associations, professional societies, and universities. Estimates of the current manpower situation in the 11 major occupational categories in the report were obtained through reviews or surveys of employers, professional associations, and graduates of schools of public health. In addition to analyses of the number of degrees awarded in each field, and of

Table 1

Estimated Supply of and Requirements for
Selected Categories of Professional Health Manpower

Professionals with Master's Level Training or Higher[1]

Occupational Category	Base Year Supply (1970 unless specified)	1980 Supply, Assuming		Possible 1980 Require-ments[3]
		Constant School Output[2]	Reduced School Output[2]	
Environmental Health	2,200	4,300	3,800	5,000
Epidemiology	1,000	1,800	1,500	2,000
Health Education	2,000	3,600	3,100	6,000
Health Services Administration	8,500	18,200	15,300	25,200
Health Statistics	1,100 (1971)	1,700	1,500	2,500
Maternal Health, Family Planning & Child Health	800	1,800	1,500	2,000
Mental Health	200	400	350	1,100
Public Health Dentistry	300	550	500	550
Public Health Nursing	2,500 (1968)	5,200	4,500	5,700
Public Health Nutrition	1,000	1,800	1,500	2,600
Public Health Veterinary Medicine	200	350	300	550

[1] Numbers over 1,000 are rounded to nearest 100; below 1,000, to nearest 50.

[2] "Constant school output" is based on the size of the average graduating class in the early 1970s. "Reduced school output" assumes that the Administration's proposed FY 1974 budget was implemented according to plan, resulting in a 35 percent reduction in the combined school output from the 1973/74 academic year on.

[3] The projected requirements *do not* take into consideration the continuing demands being made on American schools of public health to train foreign students in connection with the U.S. foreign assistance program, and the requirements of the World Health Organization. Foreign student enrollments have averaged over 15 percent in recent years.

where and how these professionals are employed, other indicators, such as membership of professional societies, were used to determine the numbers of individuals currently employed in the various specialties.

Projections of supply were made by extrapolating trends in the annual numbers of graduates from schools of public health and other educational institutions granting advanced degrees in the specialties over the past 10 years, corrected for recent changes in enrollment policies where appropriate. Loss rates for new graduates and for the existing stock of public health manpower were made on the basis of observations of similar occupations. With regard to demand, where reasonable projections had been developed by government agencies or professional societies, these were used. Where adequate demand projections did not exist, these were developed, taking into account such factors as vacancy rates for public health manpower in government and private agencies, reasonable staffing standards appropriate to the various types of public health institutions under consideration, and probable trends in government policies regarding the expansion of health activities.

The study indicates that over the next decade the greatest relative increases in public health manpower requirements will occur in mental health, health education, and health services administration. Most other subspecialties are expected at the very least to double their current manpower needs by 1980. The underlying rationale for the projections in these categories in terms of their expected roles and functions is briefly outlined below:

Environmental Health Requirements in this area are expected to double by 1980. It is apparent that man's interaction with his environment has produced an ominous potential for harm, and that the public expects to be protected. In the future, more research and planning, the clarification of jurisdictional responsibilities, and larger, more effective field programs will clearly be needed, all of which will require a significant increase in the numbers of professional environmental health personnel.

Epidemiology Requirements are expected to double. This may be an underestimate of needs, as personnel with training in epidemiology will be used in health planning and the surveillance of medical care as well as other health care services. Many large hospitals and medical centers are beginning to employ full-time epidemiologists. The growing concern with occupational health and safety, and the effects of pollution, together with the growing appreciation of the role of epidemiologic studies in uncovering the etiology and predisposing factors of chronic disease have already increased the demand for epidemiologists and will continue to do so.

Health Education   Requirements are expected to triple. We are entering a new period in which community health education and health promotion will occupy a central rather than a peripheral position. New programs to control cigarette smoking, alcohol, and other addictions, as well as hypertension, coronary heart disease, and cancer, rely heavily on health education as a major approach to achieving behavioral change in the interest of disease prevention and control.

Health Services Administration   Requirements are expected to triple. The development of federal policies with respect to health services will play a major part in determining the need for health administrators. Some of the new programs already being implemented have been referred to earlier in this chapter. These, plus the expected national health insurance legislation will require additional trained manpower for management and administration.

Health and Vital Statistics   Requirements are expected to double. This estimate of requirements may be too modest in view of the recent increase in use of quantitative approaches to the study and evaluation of medical care programs and services. In addition, environmental health programs will require more statisticians in such areas as air and water pollution, toxicology, food production and control, and land use planning.

Maternal Health, Family Planning, and Child Health   Requirements are expected to more than double. It might be assumed that the demand for specialists in this field would decrease because of the declining birth rate. However, there has been a new appreciation of unmet needs, and opportunities for effective intervention in such areas as nutrition and developmental disabilities. In addition there is a serious lack of comprehensive health services for many children, particularly in rural areas and the inner cities. All this is reflected in an expansion of support for categorical programs for these purposes.

Mental Health   Requirements are expected to increase 550 percent. In psychiatric hospitals, community mental health centers, and in other organized programs in this field, the prevailing pattern is to utilize clinicians (physicians, psychologists, social workers) as directors. Very few have had formal education in health services administration. Continued prominence of the need for mental health services, and changes in the cost and manner of delivery of such services are producing an awareness of the need for personnel with competence in planning, organizing, and evaluating these services. Though it is likely that a clinical background will continue to be required for these positions, people with the additional specialized knowledge and skills for this role will be in greater demand.

Public Health Dentistry   Estimated requirements will nearly double. These estimates are based on the increasing attention being given to preventive dentistry for children as a responsibility of public health agencies, and the fact that insurance programs have begun to include dental services in their coverage.

Public Health Nursing   Estimated requirements will more than double. Though changing public health problems and programs have produced some uncertainty about the definition of "public health nursing" for the future, the role of nursing in the community has gained prominence. The orientation, knowledge, and skills of traditional public health nursing are being adapted to preventive and management programs for such chronic diseases as cancer, hypertension, and coronary heart disease. The need for public health nursing supervision of family health workers employed by neighborhood health centers, and the growth of organized home care programs also contribute to the demand.

Public Health Nutrition   Estimated needs will more than double. Community nutrition programs are concerned with ensuring that everyone has an adequate and balanced diet—a continuing and serious problem for the poor and many of the aged. In addition, the role of nutrition in the prevention and treatment of a number of important diseases, such as hypertension, coronary heart disease, and certain developmental disabilities, is becoming clearer. Technological and merchandising developments in the food industry and the propensity for food faddism have a profound influence on health. Public programs to deal with these problems are expanding.

Public Health Veterinary Medicine Requirements are expected to more than double. The scope of veterinary public health has been expanding from just dealing with diseases transmitted from animals to man, and now includes wide participation in epidemiologic studies and in studies evaluating the effects of food additives, drugs, and environmental contaminants. In carrying out their responsibilities, veterinarians function in federal, state, and local agencies.

Comment

There will, of course, be differences in the level of responsibility and function to be assumed by personnel in each of these categories, and the educational system must take this into account. The numbers needed in each category do not refer to a single type of graduate to be educated in a single way. Educational programs must clearly recognize the level of performance their graduates are expected to achieve and adjust the curriculum accordingly.

The Commission's conviction that large numbers of people will need to be trained for activity in the field is not meant to encourage the indiscriminate expansion of educational programs. The use of new types of personnel, to assume less complex tasks and functions under the supervision of personnel trained at the graduate level, might be one way of meeting some of the manpower need.

However, the responsibility for the education of personnel for public health does not end with the preparation of new entrants into the field. Those already working in positions have a continuing need for programs of education to maintain and upgrade their knowledge and skills. For others, previous education needs supplementation so they can deal effectively with changing responsibilities. This highlights the importance of inservice and continuing education programs as a joint responsibility of health agencies and the academic community.

Shortly after World War II, George Perrott, Chairman of the Public Health Service Committee on Postwar Training, wrote that there was a need to "get statistics on the number and types of public health personnel to be trained; and watch the statistics on the

capacity of our schools of public health and other educational institutions to train them . . ." (Perrott, 1945:1155).

We believe that this statement holds true today. The nation still
needs a continuing program for the systematic collection and monitoring of data on the current and projected balance between the
supply of, and need for, public health manpower. This monitoring
is done in many other fields. Such a system would provide information on the nature of the pool of applicants, training categories,
and educational programs. It could provide a basis for discussion
on the best location of centers for advanced training, sites of
new educational programs, and curricular emphasis based on
service needs and employment opportunities. The responsibility for
generating and overseeing such a surveillance system should be
assumed by the federal government and shared with universities and
relevant professional organizations.

Recommendation

2. *A national program to monitor systematically the needs for, and
supply of, public health manpower is crucial to effective planning of
education for the field. Such a program should be developed and
conducted by the Department of Health, Education, and Welfare,
in continuous cooperation with universities, relevant professional
organizations, and public health agencies.*

5. The Knowledge Base
For Public Health

The primary goal of public health programs, to protect, preserve, and improve the health of the people, is a complex one. Its achievement depends, in the first instance, upon the basic knowledge and available technologies which, when systematically and appropriately applied to populations and communities, will produce maximum reduction of sickness, disability, and death. Of course, the nature and extent of the knowledge and technologies change with time and are not at a uniform level for all public health problems.

Evolution

Public health as a distinct practice, requiring special training and knowledge, is a relatively recent phenomenon. By the end of the eighteenth century, the increasing urbanization which accompanied the industrial revolution had exacerbated the problems of communicable disease. Devastating epidemics of cholera, smallpox, and typhoid took a high toll in lives, and were seen as interfering greatly with commerce and the smooth functioning of the body politic. By 1779 there was a growing interest in what Johann Peter Frank, Director General of Public Health of Austrian Lombardy—considered by many to be the father of the modern public health movement—described as:

> ". . . a defensive art . . . whereby human beings and their animal assistants can be protected against the disadvantageous consequences of crowding too thickly upon the ground; and especially it is an art for the promotion of their bodily weal in such a way that, without suffering from an overplus of physical evils, they

may defer to the latest possible term the fate to which, in the end, they must all succumb." (Quoted by Sigerist, 1956)

During the nineteenth century, knowledge was accumulating that would provide the means to control some communicable diseases. Vaccination against smallpox had been demonstrated by Jenner in 1798; by 1840 the British Government was providing free vaccination, and in 1867 this first immunization procedure was made compulsory. The work of Pasteur and Koch, in the middle of the century, marked the beginning of the golden age of bacteriology which quickly produced positive results in the control of water- and milk-borne diseases. Snow's classic epidemiologic study of the transmission of cholera through one of London's private water systems was yet another landmark in the conquest of epidemic disease through environmental control.

The scientific advances created a need in many western countries for a cadre of people capable of implementing this new knowledge. In the United States, many individual states established boards of health, responsible for protecting communities against communicable disease. This was to be done through the provision of sanitary water supplies, safe methods of waste disposal, supervision of the hygiene of food and milk, public laboratory services, and involvement of private physicians in communicable disease control procedures. However, death rates from epidemic disease remained high, and a common complaint at the time was the lack of programs for specialized training of professional public health personnel. Hermann Biggs, later the General Medical Officer of the New York City Health Department, wrote in 1898:

"There is everywhere lacking the presence of intelligent, thoroughly trained sanitary officers, because there are no provisions in this country for the education of men in matters of public health. The knowledge required for the intelligent discharge of the duties of medical officers of health is broad, comprehensive and entirely unlike that required for a medical advisor. There is, so far as I am aware, no place in this country where the complete training required can be obtained." (Biggs, 1898:44–50)

Scattered courses and programs were offered at various universities in the United States during the first decade of the twentieth century, but none of these provided a complete curriculum for public health practitioners. There was general agreement among the leaders at the time on who should be trained and what they should be trained for. Physicians, aiming at careers as health officers, needed instruction in sanitary engineering, vital statistics, public health law, the control of communicable diseases, and laboratory procedures for public health.

Milton Rosenau of Harvard, the first full-time professor in preventive medicine and public health in the United States, explained in 1913 both why physicians needed special training for public health work and what that training should be.

"It is now recognized that the orthodox training leading to the degree of M.D. does not necessarily fit a man for the position of health officer. The average practitioner learns very little concerning vital statistics, sanitary engineering, water purification, sewage disposal, disinfection, forensic medicine, and the making and breaking of health laws. The public health officer looks upon disease in the large, and is less interested in the individual case, which is the chief concern of the practicing physician. The health officer looks upon disease with an eye to preventing its spreading —in order to do so he must know its mode of transmission. The practicing physician looks upon disease with a view to affording relief or cure, and his principal interest, therefore, is in diagnosis and treatment. The public health officer must also be a specialist . . ." (Rosenau, 1913:29)

The Welch-Rose Report

In response to these and other articulations of need, the General Education Board, founded by John D. Rockefeller to improve education in the United States, called a conference in 1914 to consider professional training for public health work. Nineteen leaders in education, medicine, and public health attended in New York City and came to substantial agreement on the following points: 1. Adequately trained personnel was a fundamental health need. 2. A distinct contribution toward this could be made by establishing a school of public health of high standards. 3. Such a school should be closely affiliated with a university and its medical school. 4. It should be organized as a separate entity with an institute of hygiene as its nucleus.

William Welch and Wickliffe Rose were asked to formulate a plan for such a school, and in 1916 they presented a report which has greatly influenced the development of public health teaching since that time. Welch and Rose presented plans for an Institute of Hygiene to train those ". . . who expect to devote their lives to health work," including administrative officials, health officers, higher technical experts (statisticians, sanitary engineers, chemists, bacteriologists, and epidemiologists), inspectors (food, school, etc.), and nurses. They suggested that the majority of candidates would be physicians, but that others should be admitted to the institute.

> "When one considers the many points of contact between the modern social welfare movement and the public health movement, and to what extent social and economic factors enter into questions of public health, it is clear that an institute of hygiene must take full cognizance of such factors and that students of social science should profit by certain opportunities in the institute, as well as students of hygiene by training in social science and social work." (Welch and Rose, 1916a:415)

The objectives were stated to be:

> ". . . the cultivation of hygiene as a science, the development of the spirit of investigation and the advancement of knowledge, the practical task of preparing candidates for public health positions and the instruction of medical students and physicians in practice in the principles of hygiene and preventive medicine." (Welch and Rose, 1916a:415)

Thus, when plans for higher education for public health were first formulated, public health was recognized as part of a broad social movement, although the goals were perceived as the training of physicians and others in the principles of hygiene and preventive medicine. While questions of social policy were not specifically approached in the recommended curriculum, Welch and Rose indicated that they could not be ignored. They did recommend, in discussing the connection with the university, that the department of sociology be involved.

Johns Hopkins University quickly undertook to implement these recommendations and established its School of Hygiene and Public Health in 1916. As Welch and Rose predicted, this quickly stimulated the formation of similar programs. By 1922, Yale, Columbia, Harvard, and Michigan had all started special programs for career training in public health.

Expanding the Curriculum

Although the new schools of public health concentrated on the training of physicians, the activities of health departments were expanding with the consequent use of other people from an increasing number of other fields. The discovery of vitamins and their effect on health, for example, had stimulated an interest in nutrition, and nutritionists were first employed by health departments in 1917.

By 1922, when the American Medical Association recommended periodic health examinations, the need for individual participation in health protection and disease prevention was acknowledged. Skilled people were required to motivate the public and involve it in personal health activities, and in that same year a separate section of health educators was established in the American Public Health Association.

Public health practitioners soon expanded their areas of interest to include major questions of social policy. The stock market crash of 1929 and the economic depression which followed, served to stimulate broader interest in public health. This quickly produced a widespread concern with poverty and other social factors, and their effects on disease patterns. Although this may have appeared to be a new development, in fact it was a rediscovery of one of the oldest themes of public health. In 1849, in his first annual report as health officer of London, John Simon wrote:

". . . no sanitary system can be adequate to the requirements of the time, or can cure those radical evils which infect the under-framework of society, unless the importance be distinctly recognized, and the duty manfully undertaken, of improving the social condition of the poor." (Quoted in Winslow, 1948:173)

In its broadest sense this can be interpreted as dealing with all aspects of the living conditions of poor people, rather than narrowly restricting concern to known health hazards. In 1937, almost a century later, Joseph Mountin picked up the banner and condemned the

". . . hesitancy of health officers to participate in the housing movement because epidemiologists fail to find evidence of direct causal relationship between housing and health . . . It seems to me that people who call themselves health workers should go beyond disease and into the broader fields of human comfort and vitality." (Quoted in Winslow, 1937:35–45)

If the practice of public health had begun with the relatively limited goal of controlling communicable disease, by the 1930s the objectives of public health philosophers in this country had grown immeasurably. The responsibilities of society, as represented by official government agencies, were correspondingly viewed as broader and more comprehensive. In 1935, Edgar Sydenstricker wrote on *The Changing Concept of Public Health.*

"Society has a basic responsibility for assuring, to all of its members, healthful conditions of housing and living, a reasonable degree of economic security, proper facilities for curative and preventive medicine, and adequate medical care—in fact the control, so far as means are known to science, of all the environmental factors that affect physical and mental wellbeing." (Sydenstricker, 1935:30)

Broad objectives and responsibilities require large and powerful organizations to carry them out. Local and state boards of health had neither the resources nor the personnel to begin to control "all the environmental factors that affect physical and mental wellbeing," and during the 1930s the federal government became significantly involved in state programs. Under the Social Security Act of 1935, grants-in-aid were made available to the states for general public health purposes, for maternal and child hygiene, and for the care of crippled children. This commitment of federal funds brought with it the establishment and implementation of federal standards and requirements.

Although the total mobilization for World War II which ended the 1930s brought with it almost full employment and a diminishing of concern with the ill-effects of poverty, it did not decrease the involvement of the federal government in public health services. George Rosen wrote later that:

> "The modern conception that the national government is responsible for the health of the people is but a natural extension of the previous view where the local community provided for such needs. As the center of gravity has moved from the small political unit to the larger one, this has had its effect on the provision of health services. By and large, the trend today is for the national health agency to wield the greatest influence in endeavoring to relieve those notorious obstacles to human improvement, the five giants of Lord Beveridge; want, disease, ignorance, squalor, and idleness. Most recently, in fact, this trend had moved beyond the national community to the world community with the creation of the World Health Organization."
> (Rosen, 1958:468)

This shift in the center of public health responsibility from local to national organization required the development of ever-larger and more complicated administrative structures. The lone physician health officer was rapidly becoming an anachronism, and the modern public health official needed new and expanded training for new and expanded duties. In a study of schools of public health made in the early 1950s, Leonard S. Rosenfeld observed the responsiveness of the schools to the changes in public health practice.

> "All heads of departments of public health administration have found that the increasing scope of public health programs has changed the concept of training needs. A few years ago, health departments were concerned primarily with problems of environmental sanitation and communicable disease control. Now their

fields of activity include chronic disease and the provision of direct personal health services to individuals. As a consequence, the basic principles of public health practice and administration are emphasized in the courses at schools of public health to a greater extent than was true a few years ago." (Rosenfeld et al., 1953:29.)

After World War II the teaching content in higher education for public health was similarly adjusted in response to changes in the field. Many new areas were added and the emphasis was shifted.

To take one example, environmental health activities had centered on food safety (especially milk), purification of water supplies, and safe sewage disposal, and hence were described as sanitation activities. After the war, technologic advances opened the way for the use of new chemical agents in vector control. Worldwide programs, using DDT for malaria eradication, for example, created a need for people trained either in international health, pesticide use, or both. Later, as the harmful effects of these new chemicals became apparent, there was a new need for people who could understand and deal with the problems posed by these manmade hazards. In the immediate postwar years, environmental hazards were not accorded high priority because the battle for environmental sanitation was considered to have been won. But 20 years later the emphasis again reverted to what is now termed environmental health. This new and larger field:

". . . covers at least the following: water supply; wastewater engineering and water pollution control; solidwaste collection and disposal; control of disease vectors; air pollution control; environmental radiation control; industrial hygiene and toxicology; noise control; prevention of motor vehicle accidents; urban planning; architecture; and preventive occupational, and aerospace medicine." (World Health Organization, 1967a:8)

Today, environmental health activities are considered too complicated to be carried out by any single professional. The environmental health specialist must be capable of integrating a range of social and physical sciences to accomplish a desired end. In 1967, the

World Health Organization Expert Committee on the Education of
Engineers in Environmental Health stated:

> "Those who are educated in environmental health engineering
> in the coming years will spend much of their professional lives
> in planning so as to avoid lowering the quality of the environment
> and prevent environmental hazards. In doing so, they will work
> with economists, technicians, politicians, physicians, bankers and
> journalists. The expert in environmental health must be able to
> advise on the location of new cities and power plants; on the
> extent to which a fertile basin can be built up commercially and
> residentially; on the type of waste disposal that a new industry,
> factory, or crop will require; on the type of engine that can be
> used as the prime mover in a transport system; and on which
> indigenous materials are suitable for home construction and
> which must be improved . . . However successful an expert may
> be in devising a solution to a particular problem in a given area,
> he must always be prepared to find that such a solution is in-
> appropriate for another area or another problem." (World
> Health Organization, 1967b:7)

Over the past 30 years, many other special public health programs have been developed in response to perceived needs. These
include programs for the control of cancer, heart disease, or other
chronic diseases; mental health programs; alcoholism and drug
addiction programs; population control and family planning; and
medical care organization. The curriculum of higher education for
public health has changed and will continue to change as the health
problems of the nation themselves change in their nature or intensity.
This organic development of the public health curriculum was
described more than 30 years ago by Thomas Parran, Surgeon General of the United States Public Health Service, when he said:

> "The evolution of public health teaching in this country has
> reflected the expanding concept of its practice. Originally, health
> departments were concerned primarily with the control of acute
> communicable diseases. As a result, emphasis was given to this
> sphere of health teaching. With the great expansion of activities
> in connection with maternal and child health, industrial hygiene

and venereal disease control, special emphasis has been given to training leaders in these disciplines. The development of programs by health departments in medical nutrition, in mental hygiene, in health education, and in hospital administration likewise has resulted in emphasis upon the teaching of the public health aspects of these subjects. Problems of medical administration—or what may be described as social medicine—already face us and are likely to grow. As a result of the subdivision of the public health profession into its many branches some of which I have enumerated, it is highly desirable to expand curricula to meet or even to anticipate the need." (Parran, 1943–44:12)

Present Status

While acknowledging that the content of public health curricula must alter to meet and anticipate changing problems and needs in the community, it is important to recognize that there is a core of public health knowledge that can be drawn upon and can supply the fundamental basis for attacking these problems. Though, of course, modifications and additions take place as the result of research and demonstrations, the approach and basic framework remain the same.

For many years it has been assumed by many people that public health is no more than a series of related skills which are applied in a societal context. According to this conception, knowledge is borrowed from different fields as necessary, but does not constitute a coherent whole. As Welch and Rose wrote:

"Unity is to be found rather in the end to be accomplished—the preservation and improvement of health—than in the means essential to that end." (Welch and Rose, 1916a:415)

This Commission finds, however, that there is a knowledge base for public health which can be codified and which serves to achieve ". . . the end to be accomplished." It is composed of content areas which can be divided into two groups.

The first includes three elements, central and generic to public health, which flourish best in a public health setting. These are: 1. the measurement and analytic sciences of epidemiology and biostatistics; 2. social policy and the history and philosophy of public health; 3. the principles and practice of management and organization for public health.

The second group consists of a group of cognate disciplines which are, in various combinations, often fundamental to the understanding of public health problems. These disciplines develop most often and usually most favorably under auspices other than public health. However, this does not lessen their importance or ability to contribute to the understanding and solution of public health problems. A brief overview of both of these content groups is given below to clarify the Commission's view of the foundation of higher education for public health.

Fields of Knowledge
Generic to Public Health

The Measurement and Analytic Sciences: Epidemiology and Biostatistics

A definitive characteristic of public health is its approach to the health problems of communities and populations. To the clinician, the patient is the individual; to the public health professional, the client is the entire community. As a result of its social or group orientation, public health relies heavily on specialized methods of quantitative analysis. While the clinician is concerned with appraising the nature and severity of each patient's illness, the public health professional wants to know which people have become ill, why, when, and in what circumstances. The basic techniques for measuring and evaluating community-wide health problems are those of epidemiology and biostatistics, the sciences of "social (or health) arithmetic."

Epidemiology Epidemiology is the science devoted to the systematic study of the natural history of disease—its distribution in populations and the factors which determine distribution. Because it is concerned with which portion of the population becomes ill and which does not, and what preventable risk factors are present in the community, epidemiology is the basic science of public health work and of preventive medicine. It is the intelligence arm of the public health program, determining which diseases and disabilities are frequent, which rare; which are increasing in frequency, which are disappearing from the population either through unpremeditated forces or as the result of planned disease control programs; and which diseases are quiescent yet capable of affecting an unprotected population. Through its systematic studies of morbidity and mortality, epidemiology often is the key element in the search for prevention of disability and premature death. Its methods are always indispensable when appraising the degree of success of any health program.

In its descriptive role, epidemiology makes use of statistical methods to determine morbidity and mortality rates such as prevalence, incidence, case fatality rates, and to estimate risks of developing a specific disease or of dying In its analytic phase, it utilizes a variety of techniques to examine and evaluate a wide range of data which elucidate disease and disability in terms of predisposing, precipitating, and prolonging causes. These data include population characteristics, identifiable agents (biologic and nonbiologic), and environmental factors producing human disease and disability. As a constructive and diagnostic discipline, epidemiology identifies specific foci for further exploration and intervention, and suggests specific avenues for further study.

But epidemiology is more than the accumulated knowledge about the distribution of a particular disease and the factors affecting its occurrence in the population at any one time; it also delineates the chains of inference based upon these facts and other relevant facts about that disease and that population. These chains of inference or hypotheses are an integral part of the epidemiology of today. False inferences are refuted by later experience; sound inferences foretell the epidemiologic knowledge of tomorrow.

Epidemiologic techniques are used to trace the causes of specific diseases and to provide a framework for comparative studies of group health behavior with regard to chronic problems such as alcoholism, smoking, and obesity. In recent decades epidemiology has moved well beyond its traditional concerns with infectious diseases to embrace the study of factors influencing the occurrence of chronic illness, accidental death and disability, and occupational and environmental diseases. Psychological and social factors have been added to biologic and physical factors as foci of investigation. In essence, epidemiology represents both a methodologic and a descriptive approach to definition of the agent-host-environment inter-relationship which determines the collective health of populations.

Recently, epidemiology has been recognized to be crucial to the planning and evaluation of medical care and other health programs because of the contribution it can make to the development of methods for program surveillance in such terms as who is being reached, with what kinds of services, with what kind of quality, and with what outcomes.

Biostatistics   Biostatistics uses statistical methodology to investigate problems in public health and medical care. In addition to collecting, analyzing, and retrieving data, designing experiments, and developing appropriate comparisons among population groups, biostatistics applies the techniques of inference and probability to the examination of biologic data. While interacting most continuously and closely with epidemiology, biostatistic interests extend into the congruent areas of vital statistics and demography, computer programming, computer systems and analysis, and program planning and evaluation. Through the continuing collaboration of epidemiologists and biostatisticians, the science and skill of designing experiments, analytic surveys, and data analysis have progressed to an advanced level. The actual work of these two types of specialists mesh so closely at times that it may be difficult for the outsider to distinguish between them. Through a fruitful working relationship, each in fact has come to learn a great deal about the other's methods and activities. Both as an arm of epidemiology and as a separate science, biostatistics serves as the major method of quantifying and analyzing health information specifically for application within public health.

Social Policy and the History and Philosophy
of Public Health

Welch and Rose (1916a:415) wrote of ". . . the many points of contact between the modern social welfare movement and the public health movement . . .", and indeed much of the impetus to develop organized approaches to protecting and restoring the health of large groups came out of a concern for the well-being of the poor. John Simon put this point most dramatically when he wrote:

> "Only because of the physical sufferings am I entitled to speak; only because pestilence is forever within the circle; only because death so largely comforts these poor orphans of civilization . . ." (Quoted in Brockington, 1954)

Social concern on the part of individuals and groups for the health of the public has been expressed throughout human history. Clearest and earliest evidence for this is to be found whenever epidemics appeared. However, an organized approach to protecting and restoring the health of large groups did not emerge until the escalating urbanization produced by the Industrial Revolution precipitated new and widespread health problems whose presence was clearly obvious to all. These negative consequences of human achievements are a dramatic early example of the often dysfunctional results of new technology and of the individual health costs of social change which foreshadowed the ecological imbalance in our own modern industrial society. The fetid, overcrowded ghettos of the industrial poor were an ideal breeding ground for infectious disease; ultimately not only social reformers but employers as well were forced to recognize the need for immediate and drastic reform of living and working conditions, in order to reduce the serious effects on health that resulted from these conditions.

It was during this period that a number of seminal attitudes for the future development of public health were first articulated:

— that the health status of populations intimately affects and is affected by its collective economic, social, industrial, and even political behavior;

— that the duty of monitoring, assessing, and improving the

health of communities should rest with a cadre of professional
health workers;

— that the state ought to assume primary organizational and
financial responsibility for the health of the poor.

While specific emphases have varied according to time and
place, in general the history of public health is the history of pragmatic attempts to apply these three basic principles to the solution
of contemporary health problems. The study of this history reveals
all of the social and political forces which play roles in the formulation of social policy on health issues. Procedures which seem commonplace today—compulsory pasteurization of milk, for example,
or compulsory immunization—were the subject of heated conflict
in the past. Slowly and unevenly, the logic of these measures over-
came strong opposition from various quarters.

The errors and failures of public health need to be identified
and understood as do the successes. Industry's effort to prevent and
control occupational health hazards has ranged from wholehearted
compliance with governmental standards and requirements to delay
and outright evasion. It is as important for public health workers to
understand the fact of failure and the reasons for it, as it is for them
to understand the need for control measures and the means of implementing them.

The study of past and current social policy, and its relationship
to public health should not be confined to the United States. An international frame of reference is especially valuable to augment the
professional perspectives in this nation and to counteract provincialism through comparative analysis. There is much to be learned, not
only from the successes and failures of international cooperation
in public health, but also from the nature of public health problems and the solutions that have been adopted both in developed
and developing countries.

New procedures, programs, and organizations in public health
are subject to similar constraints and evoke similar conflict. An
understanding of basic, and often conflicting, social values and the
way social and political compromises were achieved in the past is
necessary for effective public health progress today. A knowledge
of the ways in which social, economic, and political forces have in-

fluenced and controlled social policy is essential to a full understanding of the actual causes of some of our major health problems, and is crucial to the development of effective solutions for them. Therefore public health professionals must not only develop a commitment to organized programs to promote the health of the community, but they must understand the lessons of history so that they can apply their specific skills and knowledge in the social arena of the present.

Management and Organization for Public Health

The professional public health worker's higher education must prepare him to organize health programs in the community. To develop a public health program, one must be able to delineate clearly a set of social purposes for a defined population and to know how to locate, develop, integrate, and manage the appropriate set of resources needed to achieve those objectives. The achievement of those health objectives often requires the mobilization of some intermediate resources and the modification of the functioning of some agencies (such as housing authorities or social welfare departments) whose primary goals are not health per se.

Management of such programs involves more than the maintenance and continued administration of an organization designed to implement laws and regulations or to provide services in a routine, prescribed way. It includes the process of modifying a community's perception of, and relationship to, a particular disease or health hazard. It means setting goals, getting others to visualize and accept those goals, and knowing how to create the organization necessary to accomplish them. While interacting with these many other social forces, public health leaders and planners must be able to keep the health mission in mind and to know how to interdigitate the diverse objectives of other public administrators with their primary mission: the protection of the people's health. The characteristics of the attitude towards, and the interest in, health on the part of various sections of the population are crucial factors, as is an appreciation of the art and science of communicating with, and educating, the public.

Successful public health activity requires an ability to identify those biologic, economic, social, and political factors that must be involved, strengthened, or otherwise modified. Similarly, it is essential that important organizations and forces in our society that are pertinent to the health of the public be adequately understood. These include the health professions and traditional organizations in the health field as well as industry's attitude to social responsibility, the economy of the country or a local area, the role of individual initiative and responsibility in protecting and restoring health, and the comparison of benefits versus cost in various facets of human life. An understanding of the total societal framework which influences the system is needed to facilitate effective modification and innovation in the organization of resources and programs to meet health needs.

Fields of Knowledge
Cognate to Public Health

Several disciplines and sciences make important contributions to public health. Their substantive content, and their methods and techniques are essential to the optimal development of public health activities. They include the clinical, biomedical, environmental, and social sciences, the applied organizational techniques of management and administration, the law, and ethics.

Clinical Sciences

The clinical sciences consist of those areas of knowledge which operate through a one-to-one, practitioner-patient relationship. They comprise medicine, nursing, and dentistry, and some aspects of social work, and emphasize the empirical application of these fields to individual health problems. The scope and nature of the services they can provide to patients, and the methods and procedures which they use must be understood so that their services can be integrated into programs to meet public health objectives most effectively. The preventive, diagnostic, and curative techniques of clinical medicine can be extended to broad-based programs for finding, diagnosing, and treating specific illnesses in population groups. The new types of health professionals now being educated to provide clinical care (such as the physician's assistant, nurse-practitioner, and health aide) can also function effectively in public health settings. Finally, an understanding of the practice of the clinical sciences is essential to the establishment of systems to maintain high quality care. In essence, then, public health seeks the optimum organization of the service aspects of these sciences to achieve its goals.

Biomedical Sciences

The biomedical sciences explore the intricacies of human development and function (e.g., anatomy, physiology, biochemistry, genetics, microbiology, and pathology) in terms of both normal and abnormal physical and mental behavior. Their approach is centered on laboratory experimentation and analysis of the factors affecting human health, including pathogenic agents, developmental abnormalities, and environmental influences. These sciences not only contribute fundamental knowledge which is then applied by the health professions, but their utility for public health also lies in their ability to pinpoint the process and effects of disease which form the bases of effective control procedures.

Environmental Sciences

The environmental sciences are concerned with the relationship between the environment and human health. Environmental health specialists use basic sciences (e.g., physics, chemistry, biology) and applied sciences (engineering, urban and regional planning, and industrial toxicology) to study such problems as air and water pollution, food contamination, radiation, noise abatement, and certain other physical factors in the environment (e.g., housing, the design of highways). In addition to the traditional personnel, sanitarians and engineers, new types of professionals in environmental health are now trained in such areas as radiation control, industrial hygiene, and occupational safety.

Social Sciences

The dynamics of human social behavior—both individual and collective—cannot be understood without the knowledge to be gained from the academic disciplines of sociology, anthropology, psychology, economics, and political science. In addition they provide the operational framework for applied professional activities such as law, social work, and management in the private and public sectors—all of which influence the health of the public. Furthermore, certain elements of the behavioral sciences contribute to the knowledge which needs to be applied by the health professions.

Public health interactions with these disciplines occur at a variety of levels. Techniques of group psychology and behavioral training are directly applicable to the alteration of societal and individual health practices and, on a pragmatic level, to the education of populations in methods of personal health care. The political process affects the organization and delivery of health programs, through the development of legislation, the adoption of regulations, and their implementation. Socioeconomic conditions have repercussions on the patterns of distribution, cost, and access to medical care within specific populations. A working knowledge of the interrelationships between social forces and health programs provides the public health professional with essential elements in the frame of reference which must be used for health activities to be maximally effective.

Management Sciences

For the management and organization of health programs, the techniques, knowledge, and skills of the management sciences are, of course, fundamental. While this knowledge can readily be thought of in terms of such elements as financial management, facility and program planning, the analysis of tasks and procedures, and personnel administration, there is a matrix of professional competence which is needed for certain types of public health responsibility, much of which has been developed by the application of relevant social sciences to the problem of management. Although one can attribute much of the recent progress in this field to the theories, techniques, and insights developed by schools and departments of business and public administration, a substantial contribution continues to be made by social science departments such as economics, psychology, sociology, anthropology, and political science.

The matrix develops the characteristics of management for public service in terms of knowledge, skills, values, and behavior. Subject matter which contributes to this is an understanding of the public-social-economic context; analytic tools—both quantitative and nonquantitative; individual, group, and organizational dynamics; the analysis of public policy, and management and administrative concepts and methods (Englebert, 1974). The theory and techniques of management for private enterprises, though of course relevant to public health, need to be modified and supplemented to recognize the special nature of its public purpose and its direct accountability to the community. This is because the contributions to public health are increasingly considered to be almost completely in the public sector, regardless of the nature of the auspice of a particular individual activity. While there is no doubt that the talent for managerial responsibility is not found equally in all individuals, the management sciences have a great deal to contribute to the effectiveness of the leadership for public health programs.

Law

The relationship of law to public health has changed dramatically in the past 20 years. Probably the most significant development has been the establishment and marked expansion by federal legislation of federal roles in many health and health-related areas: Medicare and Medicaid legislation, providing payment for medical care for large sections of our population; the Occupational Safety and Health Act of 1970, mandating a safe working environment and control of potential health hazards; and the National Health Planning and Resources Development Act of 1974 which sets up a national network of more than 200 local health planning organizations. These laws have increased the expectations and entitlement of the public to more accessible, efficient, and high quality health services and have highlighted the need for greater accountability on the part of those who provide these services. Other laws dealing with the environment and environmental controls have created a new regulatory climate in this all-pervasive field.

Public health professionals need a working knowledge not only of those laws and regulations which affect health agencies and institutions, but also of the sociopolitical antecedents and health effects of such laws. Most public health authority is derived from regulatory powers. Public health professionals depend on and use federal, state, and municipal legislation, court decisions, and administrative rules, regulations, and standards, to establish and enforce specific policies. The legislative process, vested interests, and politics are inextricably involved in health policies and programs. The public health professional must therefore have some understanding of general legal principles and practices as well as of specific health laws, if he or she is to function intelligently and effectively in today's complex of legislation, organizations, and programs.

Ethics

The study of ethics needs special attention in education for public health much more than it did in the past. The applicability of ethical considerations to the preservation and protection of human life and health, whether on an individual or a mass basis, is a problem of increasing seriousness. Implicit in many of today's health problems is a confrontation between moral and other values, whether these be related to social inequalities in health care, conflicts between the control of environmental hazards and economic interests, or choices to be made about the desirability of implementing a technologic advance.

Public health is part of the effort to achieve the public welfare or common good, and public health workers need to understand that concept and how it relates to society and to their own work. More specifically, they need to think through the meaning and value of propositions or principles such as the following:

—Health is a right of all people and should not be the privilege of some.

—All people are entitled to some basic minimal acceptable levels of health protection and medical care.

—High quality care is to be assured for all people.

The study of ethics should help public health professionals understand major issues connected with their work, the principal positions taken by various groups on those issues, the presuppositions and values of those who hold each position, and finally the likely consequences of those which prevail. They must not only be prepared to participate in debate regarding these matters and be aware of all the highly sensitive issues involved, but must also be ready to take action to achieve desired aims. In public health, knowledge of, and commitment to, ethical values will be of little consequence unless professionals can embody these in their own practice, explain them cogently, and persuade others to accept them. Clearly, those individuals who accept responsibility for the health of the public must be adequately prepared to play an effective part in shaping the collective conscience of the nation.

Interdependence of Public Health and Cognate Fields of Knowledge

The relationship of cognate fields and disciplines to public health is not simply one of contributing to public health understanding and activity. The relationship is reciprocal: the fields of theory and practice cognate to public health are improved, deepened, and refined by their involvement with public health problems and programs.

Microbiology is a good example of a biomedical science which has had an extremely important influence on public health and continues to provide essential knowledge to this field. Although most departments of microbiology are located in medical schools, their acquisition of new knowledge has been influenced by involvement in public health activities. The study of the occurrence of epidemics and the recognition of new diseases produced by various types of pathogenic organisms has furthered the development of microbiology as a biomedical science through the lessons learned in the public health application of its knowledge and techniques. Whereas both the earlier and continuing emphases in bacteriology were, and still are on the prevention and control of disease involving the science of immunology, recent developments have provided an impetus for the use of microbiology in fundamental studies of genetics—providing new information of significance to public health.

Similar examples of this two-way street are to be found in the social sciences. Talcott Parsons's studies of the physician-patient relationship in Boston in the 1930s and 1940s (Parsons, 1951) have had significant implications for the development of role theory in American sociology. In particular, Parsons emphasized the asymmetry and complementary nature of the contributions of each to the role relationship, and the extent to which the entire interaction rested upon a core of shared values. Later, Parsons and Fox (1952) elaborated these ideas in analyzing both the psychotherapeutic process and parent-child interaction in the American family. Thus the investigation of a health problem has had important consequences for theoretical advances in two key areas of sociology: role theory and socialization theory. More generally, much research in chronic disease bears on the theoretical understanding of "stress" in social psychology, as in the influence of important changes in individual life-space and life-style on the development of certain diseases and their symptoms.

Applying the Knowledge Base
to Public Health Teaching

It may surprise some people that some of the most important problems or activities of public health are not mentioned in this catalogue of the elements of the knowledge base. They might ask, for example, "What about environmental health?" Or "where is infectious disease control," "mental health", "nutrition", "population?"

The Commission believes it is important to differentiate between the sources that the public health curriculum must draw upon and the programs to which that curriculum is to be applied. No matter what the practical problem, the knowledge base provides the basic information, understanding, and methods necessary to deal with that problem.

A curriculum for practice and research in environmental health will of necessity draw heavily upon the environmental sciences. The basic sciences of physics, chemistry, biology, and pathology are needed to identify polluting or hazardous agents and to pinpoint their physiologic effects. Applied sciences, such as engineering, are essential in the design of industrial processes, highways, and cities to give appropriate attention to public health needs. But any program of education for environmental health must also bring in much information from the social and behavioral sciences. Environmental health specialists must be aware of economic pressures and costs in control activities, and psychologic factors may be as important as physical ones in some instances (motivating workers to wear safety gear or automobile drivers to avoid accidents). The three basic elements central to public health will still be essential: epidemiology and biostatistics to identify and measure the environmental hazards, public health management principles for the organization of environmental control programs, and the history of public health to illuminate the present by examples from the past. All of these disciplines, appropriately put together, will make up an effective teaching program in environmental health.

Similarly for other fields. The traditional activity of infectious disease control depends heavily upon biostatistics and epidemiology, health administration, the clinical sciences, and the biomedical sciences. Mental health relies on these with a still greater input from the clinical, social, and behavioral sciences.

The study of nutrition synthesizes knowledge from various sciences—clinical, biologic, social, and environmental. The epidemiologic investigations of deficiency diseases, nutritional practices in various nations and among specific populations, and nutrition-related diseases such as the cardiovascular diseases, obesity, and osteoporosis, point to important opportunities for prevention and intervention. The socioeconomic and political aspects of nutrition, food safety, and the role of regulatory agencies in public policy, and the techniques of health promotion and specific goals of preventive nutrition programs should also be understood.

In the past several decades the accelerating rate of population growth has emerged as one of the leading threats to the health and welfare of the human race. In addition to epidemiology, demography, knowledge of maternal and child health practice, and the management sciences, the social sciences—economics, sociology, anthropology—and religion are vital to an understanding of the nature and dimension of the population problems and to provide a basis for policy and program development.

The Commission has classified certain elements of the knowledge base as being generic to public health because their major development has taken place under public health auspices. This formulation does not relieve the programs of higher education in public health from the responsibility of seeing to it that the needed elements from the fields of knowledge cognate to public health are incorporated in the curriculum at a high level of quality.

There are many different types of specialists in public health carrying out responsibilities in organized programs in terms of the substantive content of their specialty and the level of their duties in the programs in which they work. The mix of knowledge that they need to have will vary depending upon the nature of their responsibilities. Thus, the educational experience for each student will be related to the student's own background and career goal, but will draw from the knowledge base in the appropriate manner. All must include the three central elements of the knowledge base for public health as well as selected portions of the different cognate disciplines suitable to the student's needs.

Recommendation

3. In order to produce professional personnel with the appropriate knowledge, skills, and perspective so that they might deal effectively with the new challenges in public health, all institutions providing higher education for public health should build their educational programs on the unique knowledge base for public health. This combines the three elements central and generic to public health with content from many related fields such as medicine and other patient care disciplines; economics, political science, and sociology; biology and the physical sciences. The elements central to public health are the measurement and analytic sciences of epidemiology and biostatistics; social policy and the history and philosophy of public health; and the principles of management and organization for public health. This knowledge base may be modified and expanded with changes in the nature and scope of health problems and the techniques used to deal with them, but an appropriate mix of its central elements with selected related fields is crucial to the effectiveness of any program of higher education for public health.

6. Current Efforts
in Higher Education
for Public Health

Higher education for public health is now provided in several different academic settings, namely schools of public health, programs in other graduate schools of the university, and baccalaureate programs. These have all developed independently of each other and in response to manpower needs in the field.

Schools of Public Health

Following the establishment of the first school of public health at Johns Hopkins University in 1916, three other such schools or institutes were established by 1922 at Yale, Harvard, and Columbia Universities. These schools were small and their programs concentrated chiefly on training physicians and engineers. The fundamental core of their instruction was biostatistics, epidemiology, public health administration, and sanitary engineering.

Though the United States started special programs of education for public health activity later than Europe, once these programs were actually begun they became pre-eminent. With some notable exceptions, many of the world's public health leaders of the last four or five decades were trained in American schools of public health, particularly the early ones.

By 1941 four state universities had entered the field with formally organized schools—Michigan, Minnesota, North Carolina, and California at Berkeley. The Social Security Act of 1935 authorized grants-in-aid to the states for certain public health programs, provided that the specified minimum qualifications for the professional public health personnel in state and local agencies were met. Substantial funds were available if the states trained people to organize and administer health and welfare programs. Federal financial aid was given to a number of universities to establish or expand training courses.

In 1946 the American Public Health Association developed an accreditation program for schools of public health (Committee on Professional Education, American Public Health Association, 1942). New schools continued to spring up, at the Universities of California at Los Angeles, Puerto Rico, Tulane, and Pittsburgh. By 1960 there were 12 schools of public health in the United States, six at private and six at public universities. Following this slow growth over four decades, eight additional schools have been founded since 1965. One of these schools, Loma Linda University, is private. All the others are located at state universities in Hawaii, Oklahoma, Texas, Washington, Illinois, Massachusetts, and South Carolina. Thus, there are now 20 schools in the United States, approximately two-thirds at public universities.

One thing that differentiates schools of public health from other graduate or professional schools is that it is no longer possible to think of them as turning out one predominant type of professional. For example, in the eyes of the public and of most members of these professions, medical and law schools are places where doctors and lawyers are trained—a single type of professional person. Public health professionals represent a wide variety of backgrounds, knowledge, and skills, and the field draws people from other professions to a significant extent.

The schools of public health also differ greatly from each other. Although they all have programs in the central public health sciences, they vary widely in their emphasis on different fields and cognate disciplines. They also vary much more than do schools of law and medicine in the numbers and kinds of departments they maintain, and the ways in which these are organized. There are also large differences in the size of the faculty for each department as well as in the nature of faculty interest, skills, and areas of competence.

Many different graduate degrees are offered by these schools.

All schools offer a Master of Public Health (M.P.H.) and most offer a Master of Science (M.S.). Master's degrees are also offered in Hygiene, Health Sciences, Hospital Administration, and a number of other specialty fields. Doctoral programs, offered in all schools except those most recently established, confer doctorates in Philosophy (Ph.D.), Public Health (Dr. P.H.), or Science (D.Sc.).

The length of the educational program varies from less than a year for a master's program in some schools to over two years in others. This represents an accommodation to the varied backgrounds of students and the scope of curriculum requirements. Doctoral programs, of course, require longer study.

The increase in the number of schools has been outpaced by the growth in enrollment in all types of programs. In the 14 years from 1958 to 1972, enrollment quadrupled from 1,230 to 4,802. In the last four years of that period, the growth in enrollment was 40 percent (Breslow, 1973). Another illustration of this growth is that the total number of graduate degrees (master's and doctoral) awarded in 1974 was 2,510, having almost doubled since 1968 when the comparable figure was 1,337 (Association of Schools of Public Health, 1975). Though most of these were at the master's level, the number of doctorates awarded by schools of public health rose steadily from 36, or 5 percent of the total in 1960, to 178, or more than 10 percent in 1970 (Richardson, 1973a). In 1974, 197 doctorates were awarded. However, this represented only 8 percent of the degrees awarded because of the larger increase in the number of master's level students (Association of Schools of Public Health, 1975).

This increase reflects a perceived need by students and health agencies which they expect will be met by the schools. The pressure upon the schools to admit more students continues unabated. There is evidence that the academic quality of the applicants is improving. The graduates of these programs also seem to have no difficulty securing employment in the field.

The schools vary greatly in the size of the student body. In 1974 the size of the graduating class varied from 39 to 283. The range of difference in size of student body among the well-established schools is approximately fivefold. This difference is not related to the length of time the school has been in existence. An examination of the rate of growth for those schools that were well established by 1960 shows that between 1960 and 1970 the number of graduates tripled at some schools, such as North Carolina and Puerto Rico, and doubled at others, such as Yale and Johns Hopkins (Richardson, 1973a). Others showed much less growth. In 1974, 12 schools awarded 83 percent of the degrees.

Over the years major changes have taken place in the nature of the student body in these schools. As mentioned previously, graduate education in public health was originally intended primarily for physicians and engineers. Recognizing that many other professions and disciplines were needed, the schools of public health were, by the 1960s, enrolling students from as many as 22 widely disparate specified professional groups. These included dentists, social workers, teachers, administrators, and laboratory scientists.

Until the past decade or so, most students were those who already had their basic professional preparation, such as medicine, dentistry, or nursing; and many of these already had field experience in public health. They came for the graduate education they needed in order to apply their profession most effectively in public health programs. To an extent this is still the case, and a few schools continue to concentrate on providing this kind of specialized training. However, entering students present a vastly different picture today than they did previously. The median age is lower, previous education is more diverse, and more students are being admitted without experience in the health field or a prior professional or graduate degree. This change offers the advantage of a potentially much larger recruitment pool for public health personnel but it represents a substantial change in policy for these schools.

Areas of Study

The expansion of the student body represents mounting enrollment in long established areas of study as well as in new programs. The central sciences, such as epidemiology and biostatistics, have continued to attract additional students, while the relative growth in applied fields, such as health services administration and maternal and child health, has been even greater. For example, in maternal and child health 300 students were enrolled in 1973, a tenfold increase in a decade (White, 1973).

In the 1960s there was a great proliferation of new, specialized programs. These quickly attracted students. They were established to develop specialized personnel as public health programs moved into new fields. Often this movement was stimulated by the availability of federal funds earmarked for a particular emphasis and focus, to meet the anticipated skilled manpower needs of newly established programs. Population and family planning, for example, came into being as a specialty program in the mid-1960s. By 1972, 800 students had been graduated with a major concentration in this area (Oakley, 1973).

An examination of student interest in major subject areas shows that between 1960 and 1970, the most popular fields of specialization were public health administration, medical care, and hospital administration, with each of these attracting approximately 14 percent of the student body. The next largest group was in health education. These fields plus environmental health, public health nursing, and epidemiology account for the interest of 60 percent of the students. Some 18 other subject areas account for the remainder (Richardson, 1973a). Table 2 sets out the wide range of specialized fields for which the schools of public health, as a group, prepare professional personnel. While all schools offer programs in the basic specialty fields, no single school offers the entire list.

Graduate Programs in Other Schools of the University

An increasing number of graduate programs now educate personnel who will devote their full time to public health. There are five specialty fields in which there are substantial numbers of graduates at the master's level from programs conducted outside schools of public health. These are health administration, nutrition, public health nursing, health education, and environmental health. In the last three, the number of graduates in recent years clearly exceeds those from schools of public health. The location of these

Table 2

**1960–1970 Graduates of Schools of Public Health
by Major Subject of Interest**

Major Subject	Total Graduates (1960–1970)	
	Number	Percentage of Total
Administrative Public Health	1715	14.5
Medical Care and Hospital Administration	1643	13.9
Health Education	1251	10.6
Environmental Health	1034	8.7
Public Health Nursing	827	7.0
Epidemiology	728	6.1
Nutrition and Biochemistry	662	5.6
Maternal and Child Health	606	5.1
Biostatistics	585	4.9
Microbiology and Laboratory Public Health	418	3.5
Tropical Medicine, Entomology, and Parasitology	367	3.1
Occupational Health	326	2.8
Dental Public Health	289	2.4
Radiological Science	241	2.0
Aerospace Medicine	218	1.8
Mental Health	197	1.7
Population Studies	168	1.4
International Health	117	1.0
Chronic Diseases	92	0.8
Veterinary Public Health	79	0.7
Behavioral and Social Sciences	78	0.7
Physiological Hygiene	52	0.4
Social Work in Public Health	40	0.3
Teaching of Preventive Medicine	16	0.1
	11851	100.0

Source: Richardson, Arthur H., Report of the Fiscal Scheme Study for the Association of Schools of Public Health. (Bureau of Manpower Education Contract NIH 71-4159.) Johns Hopkins University, May 5, 1973.

programs in the university follows the natural function of the sponsoring school or department. Thus, the public health dimensions of engineering are developed in schools of engineering, administration of health services in schools of public and/or business administration, public health nursing in schools of nursing, and health education in schools of education and communication.

It has been difficult to collect full information about all these programs because a comprehensive national listing is not maintained for each of these specialty fields. In some fields there is a recognized accreditation mechanism, and programs which are accredited can be enumerated. However, there are additional institutions offering specialty education which do not seek to have their programs reviewed for accreditation but nonetheless should be counted as contributing personnel developed at the graduate level. Further, there is evidence that employers do not distinguish between graduates of accredited and nonaccredited programs. Thus, our estimates are based on existing comparable data, with extrapolations where necessary from other sources of information.

A brief description of these educational programs in single fields follows.

Health Administration

Graduate programs in health and/or hospital administration are offered in many academic settings in addition to those in schools of public health. These include schools or departments of business administration, public administration, business and public administration, medical schools, schools of allied health, independent graduate programs and several others. There are 43 such programs in existence today (Commission on Education for Health Administration, 1975a), some of which are not accredited. Impetus for much of this development came from hospital and health service administrators who believed, for example, that expertise in the knowledge and skills of business administration was central to their field of responsibility.

The first graduate program in hospital administration was established at the University of Chicago in 1934. In the next 26 years, nine additional programs were established at other universities (Wren, 1967). Since 1960 there has been such a demand for people trained in health and/or hospital administration that in the 12 years from 1960–1972, 14 new programs were started in additional universities. Whereas up to 1960 there was a total of 3,120 graduates of these accredited programs (an average of 120 per year) at the present time there are at least 644 graduates each year (personal communication with Dr. G. Filerman, 1975).

Many of these programs, originally focusing on hospital administration only, have expanded their curriculum to make it possible for students to concentrate on general health services administration and health planning in addition to, or instead of, institutional administration. This was paralleled in the schools of public health by the development and expansion of departments and programs in hospital administration, health services administration, medical care organization and planning, in addition to, or as a replacement for, their traditional programs in public health administration.

There are indications that the number of these graduate programs will increase and that there will be further specialty development in administration of health maintenance organizations and long-term care, mental health, emergency, and ambulatory care services. Additionally, graduate programs in social work and regional and urban planning are preparing personnel in planning for human services including health services. There is reason to believe that the number of graduates from these various programs will soon exceed the number of graduates in health administration from schools of public health.

Various degrees are awarded by these graduate programs such as Master of Science (M.S.), Master of Public Administration (M.P.A.) or Master of Business Administration (M.B.A.) with a major in health, Master of Health Services Administration (M.H.S.A.), or Master of Hospital Administration (M.H.A.). Some of these programs also award doctoral degrees.

Public Health Nutrition

In 1971 there were five graduate programs in public health nutrition located outside schools of public health and they awarded 40 graduate degrees (National Center for Health Statistics, 1973c). By 1974 there were approximately 15 graduate programs which awarded 80 graduate degrees (personal communication with Dr. S. Starr, 1975). Although the schools of public health still provide most of the graduates in public health nutrition, there appears to be a trend towards expansion of education in this field elsewhere in the university. A variety of other graduate schools is involved, such as colleges of home economics, education, and human development, plus schools and departments of nutrition.

Public Health Nursing

Since World War II there has been a substantial increase in the number of nurses employed in public health agencies, reflecting a greater volume of services being rendered in the community. This growth represents much more than a reflection of the increase in the size of the population. There has also been an increase in the number of public health nurses who are educationally prepared for public health work, with larger increases in nurses who are prepared for employment as supervisors, teachers, consultants, administrators, etc. (Roberts, 1968).

For several decades most of the specialized preparation for public health nursing was available through specialized certificate or special baccalaureate programs. Since 1963, all students enrolled in a baccalaureate program in general nursing have been exposed to some public health/community nursing content in the curriculum. Though only some of these nurses go on to graduate education in public health, they are all considered to have adequate basic preparation for public health nursing to occupy staff positions in public health agencies.

The curriculum for the associate degree (junior college graduate) in nursing and in the hospital diploma programs does not provide adequate content for public health/community nursing. Graduates of these programs are not considered to be prepared for public health activity. When they are employed by public health agencies these nurses are assigned to clinical staff duties, and on-the-job training is given to bridge their gap in knowledge and skills.

In 1972 an estimated 4,183 (8 percent) of the 56,400 public health nurses employed in the United States held master's degrees (School of Public Health, University of North Carolina at Chapel Hill, 1974). According to the National League for Nursing, in 1974 there were 281 master's degrees awarded in public health nursing, approximately one-third from schools of public health and two-thirds from public health nursing programs at schools of nursing (Johnson, 1975). In that year more than 30 schools of nursing offered these graduate programs with major emphasis on the advanced training of clinical nurse specialists to work in community programs (i.e., pediatric associate, midwifery, geriatric nursing, occupational health) or to take responsibility for supervision and teaching. The schools of public health programs concentrate primarily on administration and the preparation of educators.

Health Education

There are many programs in community health education, as distinct from school health education, now being offered in various graduate programs outside the schools of public health. Most of these are located in schools of education or allied health.

One source (National Center for Health Statistics, 1973d) indicates that in 1972 there were 17 schools offering these programs. Later data (personal communication with Prof. S. K. Simonds, 1975) suggests that currently there are more than 30 of these programs. Four of these alone graduated 157 health educators in 1973. Thus, a conservative estimate would probably show more than 500 degrees conferred each year by graduate programs in community health education outside schools of public health. The number of degrees conferred by schools of public health in this field was 255 in 1974 (personal communication with R. H. McLean, 1975).

Environmental Health

In 1968 the federal government awarded grants for graduate training in environmental protection to 90 institutions which did not have schools of public health associated with them. There is no report on the number of graduates of these programs, which trained students in the environmental specialty fields of air pollution, industrial hygiene, radiation protection, solid wastes, water, and general environmental protection (Magnuson, 1971). However, for 1972–73 the Register of Environmental Engineering Graduate Programs reports that there were 59 institutions without a school of public health which awarded 585 master's degrees and 65 doctoral degrees in environmental health. It is reasonable to assume that these figures underestimate the number of graduates of environmental health programs outside schools of public health for that year.

Enrollment in these programs, as distinct from graduates, was 2,157 in the master's programs and 495 in the doctoral programs. Thus, for the same 59 institutions one would expect more than 1,000 students to receive graduate degrees in 1973–74, which indicates a substantial growth rate in these programs (Klosky, 1974).

These programs are located in technical and engineering schools, and in university departments which specialize in chemical and civil engineering and environmental sciences. The schools of public health currently award approximately 200 master's degrees each year in environmental health. Thus the major development and education of manpower for the fields takes place outside schools of public health.

Undergraduate Education

Several different programs have been developed at the undergraduate level to prepare students for specific careers in the health field, including some for public health. Much of the knowledge and techniques acquired in these programs is utilized elsewhere in the health services system as well as in public health settings. These programs have been developed at the baccalaureate level within the general arts and sciences curriculum.

Junior and Community Colleges

The network of junior and community colleges has grown tremendously over the past decade. In 1974 more than 69,000 students were enrolled in various allied health programs at this level. Most are in nursing and technical fields such as laboratory services, environmental control services, and dietary technicians (Hawthorne and Perry, 1974). These graduates are not prepared specifically for public health, but develop basic skills enabling them to work as supportive and technical staff in a variety of health agencies and medical care institutions.

Recently, associate degree programs in health administration have been developed. There were two such programs in 1967, 16 in development by 1971, and about 25 other programs planned to start over the next few years. There were 160 graduates in 1971 and this number is predicted to exceed 500 by 1980 (Kraff, 1972).

Many new courses and programs are being generated to meet

growing community health needs. As a result of its close ties with the region it serves, the junior and/or community college often attempts to respond quickly to local health manpower needs.

Colleges and Universities—Baccalaureate Level

In the past few years there has been a rapid expansion of college programs for specialty areas fundamental or congruent to public health, both in the numbers of programs and in the numbers of graduates in each program. The greatest growth has been in health administration, environmental engineering, health education, and nutrition.

The baccalaureate programs in health administration undertake to prepare entry-level personnel for departmental administration in hospitals, for administration of long-term care institutions, and for administrative support services in a variety of health agencies. In 1971 there were nine programs which graduated 108 students (Kraff, 1972). A 1973 survey identified 12 programs which awarded 170 degrees (Commission on Education for Health Administration, 1975a). Though it is not possible to verify these data precisely, an estimated 40 programs were in operation in 1975 (Filerman, 1975) in colleges and departments of arts and sciences, business, and allied health, graduating approximately 400 students; and by 1980 there will probably be some 60 programs graduating between 700 and 800 students.

In addition to the baccalaureate programs in health administration, in 1972, 58 academic institutions offered undergraduate four-year programs in environmental engineering which graduated 150 persons. These graduates function as sanitarians and environmentalists in health and environmental surveillance agencies. Approximately 25 colleges offered undergraduate programs in community health education and three times as many prepared personnel for school health education activities. There were approximately 83 recognized programs for the preparation of dietitians and nutritionists (Association of Schools of Allied Health Professions, 1971).

For some time, and until the early 1960s, schools of public health at the University of California at Berkeley, University of California at Los Angeles, University of North Carolina at Chapel Hill, University of Michigan, and University of Puerto Rico offered various programs of study leading to a baccalaureate degree, most frequently in public health nursing and in sanitary engineering. This effort gradually diminished or disappeared in these schools so that by 1973 only 3 percent of the degrees awarded were at this level (Association of Schools of Public Health, 1975). Recently there has been renewed interest in the development of programs at the baccalaureate level. The School of Public Health at the University of California at Berkeley, for example, is participating in a new program leading to a bachelor of arts with a major in health arts and sciences (Winkelstein, 1975). The University of North Carolina at Chapel Hill is planning a program for a bachelor of science in public health with a major in health administration, biostatistics, nutrition, or health education (Jain, 1975).

Education at the baccalaureate level for several categoric fields in public health has grown in response to perceived manpower needs. Academic institutions have been able to link some of these new curricula to existing programs and course offerings in political science, economics, business administration, and education. These graduates are prepared to function in a limited manner in the health field or can pursue further graduate study in their area of interest.

Discussion

There are several striking features about current efforts in higher education for public health in this country. The first is that it has become a complex enterprise of considerable size and diversity, with approximately 5,000 graduate degrees conferred each year. The second is that it is still a growth industry with the number of students and programs increasing each year, and no apparent end in sight. Third, while it has been customary to think of higher education for public health primarily in terms of those few schools established solely for that purpose, a major portion of this education—about one half the degrees—is now carried on outside the schools of public health.

The schools of public health are still the major resource for education in a number of fields. This is true of health administration and nutrition, although other programs of comparatively substantial size now exist, and indicate growth at a rapid rate. In other special and important fields of public health—epidemiology, biostatistics, occupational health, dental public health, aerospace medicine, population and family planning, and international health—these schools are the predominant or only resource. On the other hand, graduate programs in other parts of the university now prepare many more people for environmental health, public health nursing, and health education than do the schools of public health. Many schools, departments, or special curricula within the university are used for graduate education for public health. Each of these considers itself able to bring unique qualities to its academic program—either because of the academic locus of the program, or the special emphasis it has developed.

The unique quality of teaching and research programs in schools of public health is considered to be the concentration on problems of the health of populations and on disease prevention. This represents a distinct and crucial difference from the emphasis which prevails in schools of medicine, nursing, or dentistry, where the concentration is on the immediate clinical problems of individuals. Similarly, schools of business and public administration emphasize the management sciences and organizational theory upon which the effective practice of public health is dependent. The Commission believes that special qualities inherent in each type of educational setting have an appropriate role in the development of the spectrum of manpower required for public health.

Up to now, graduate programs in public health in various schools of the university have grown up without regard to how they fit into the total framework of higher education for public health. Schools of public health have also been established almost as if they were the only source of personnel for public health activity. A rational structure for the total educational effort would maximize the potential of all the different types of programs. The Commission's proposals for such a structure are the substance of the following sections of this report.

III: Rationalizing Higher Education for Public Health

7. A Rational Structure

The Commission views the diversity of efforts in higher education for public health as essentially healthy. All of the models described have contributions to make. However, the appropriate part each plays in relation to the total scheme of education must be clearly delineated if the maximum educational potential is to be realized.

The separate programs in different graduate schools chiefly prepare their graduates for entry-level or middle-management positions in the fields described in the previous chapter. The schools of public health have the faculty resources, with the potential to educate in much greater depth and to prepare graduates who are theoretically capable of assuming the broadest responsibilities for planning public health programs, participating in social policy determination, and undertaking education in public health. These schools are also preparing graduates who will function at the same level in the field as will the graduates of individual programs. This is an uneconomic and frequently dysfunctional use of the resources of the schools of public health. We believe that thought should be given to a cooperative restructuring of goals and programs among all the institutions now involved in higher education for public health.

Functions of Schools
of Public Health

The need for operating level personnel in the field is undisputed. Several state legislatures have recently responded to this need by establishing schools of public health. In Illinois, Massachusetts, and South Carolina new schools have been established within the past five years ". . . prompted by a long-standing recognition of the acute and growing need for trained public health workers . . ." (School of Public Health, University of Illinois, 1972). However, a school of public health is, and should be more than just a training ground for personnel. As Welch and Rose (1916b:666) wrote in their description of an Institute of Hygiene:

"While it is not difficult to bring together on paper a group of courses selected from the several schools and departments of the university and by the addition of a few new courses make a presentable prospectus of a school of public health, this is not the conception of such a school or institute as we believe will best fulfill the functions of developing the science and art of hygiene and training for this new profession. If the institute is to make itself felt as a constructive force it must have in it a group of scientific investigators and teachers whose absorbing interest is in developing the science of hygiene and applying it to the conservation of health.

". . . It would be a misfortune if this broader conception of the fundamental agency required for the advancement of hygienic knowledge and hygienic education should be obscured through efforts directed solely towards meeting in the readiest way existing emergencies in public health service."

For several years this "misfortune" has been occurring, partly in response to pressure from federal and state governments. Because of the pressing need for personnel for public health, government funds have been made available for the production of manpower, and the schools have naturally responded. These funds have often enabled a school or particular department to develop faculty and other resources, and thus have enriched the fabric of public health education. But we question the wisdom of perpetuating a situation which developed unplanned and which now appears to have outlived its usefulness. Certainly, in the future, state legislatures should give careful consideration to alternative means of training specific types of public health workers before they establish new schools of public health at their state universities.

Existing schools of public health should also give serious and open-minded thought to the manner in which they can contribute maximally to the field of practice and to the future of public health. The Commission believes that one way they can fulfill their potential is to concentrate their efforts on those groups of students who particularly need the unique resources of the schools. We suggest that the preparation of biostatisticians, epidemiologists, research scientists, future educators, and those who will perform executive functions in the field, is the most logical function for a school of public health.

Schools of public health are the major source of education in biostatistics and epidemiology. These schools provide the optimum combination of methodologic training and substantive content for public health biostatisticians and epidemiologists. It would be inadvisable and undesirable to attempt to shift their education to another location. They have much to gain from exposure to other elements in the knowledge base for public health, and their presence in the graduate schools serves to strengthen the teaching of the central sciences and methods of analysis which are essential and fundamental to all public health theory and practice.

Research is a fundamental part of public health and of any educational endeavor. If a school of public health is to perform its proper function of ". . . developing the science and art of hygiene and of training for this new profession . . ." it must carry on an active research program. This will contribute to the academic experience of all its students. The Commission also believes that the schools of public health should develop research scientists for the various fields of public health. Naturally, some research scientists will be developed elsewhere and work on public health projects, but the schools of public health carry major responsibility for nurturing such research.

Except in certain very specialized fields, it will also be advisable if those who will be educators in public health have some experience with the full range of the knowledge base. Although dedication to his or her own specialty is necessary for any faculty member, it is also important in public health for him or her to be able to relate this specialty to what is going on elsewhere in the field. In fact, most teachers of public health are also involved (and should be) in research activity, so there is a twofold reason for their preparation in schools of public health.

The Commission strongly believes that people who use their

public health training in positions which connote a responsibility for policy determination and program development must have an overall comprehension of the field which will enable them to set priorities, allocate resources, and plan for the future. They must have information about, and understanding of, health problems, the way in which social policy is determined and carried out, and the ethical, political, and psychological implications of both of these. They must also have many specific skills and administrative techniques at their disposal. This means that they must be offered a curriculum which encompasses all elements of the knowledge base for public health at an advanced level. At the present time the schools of public health possess the best *potential* for providing the resources and organization necessary for this task.

Those who will occupy leadership positions in some specialty of public health, such as mental health or maternal and child health, will also require the comprehensive education which a school of public health should be able to provide. In contrast to clinical medicine, where specialists at the highest level tend to concentrate on an ever-narrowing area of specialization, in public health the higher the level the greater the need for a broad knowledge of the entire field. A state director of mental health services, for example, must not only be an expert in psychiatry, but must also be able to work with other state agencies on balanced programs, to represent his program to legislators and the public, and to integrate the efforts of biostatisticians, economists, social workers, and many others. In addition to advanced work in their specialty, these leaders in special fields must be able to function within the full range of the knowledge base for public health.

Functions of Graduate Schools

The many programs in various graduate schools of the university can, and should, assume the major responsibility for training the large number of professionals who will be engaged in providing the range of clearly differentiated specialty services now necessary in public health. There are already several such fields where more students are prepared for the operating level outside schools of public health than in them. Public health nurses, health educators, and environmental health specialists are now being educated outside schools of public health in far greater numbers than in the schools. If attention is given to ensuring that the three elements of the knowledge base generic to public health are adequately represented in these programs, there is no reason to believe that graduates will not be prepared equally well as graduates of schools of public health for specialty practice in the field. Certainly, there is no indication from the field today that important differences in quality of performance can be observed in relation to where people already in the field received their training.

It is also far easier and more economic to assemble the elements needed for a graduate program in a single public health specialty than it is to develop or even maintain a first-class school of public health. The location of the specialty program in the school of its parent discipline (such as public health nursing in a nursing school or health care administration in a school of public administration) should ensure that the primary function for which the student is being prepared will be well taught. Some aspects of environmental health are dependent upon engineering solutions, for example, and are naturally developed in a school of engineering. Representatives of operating agencies could well look to these graduate programs for most of their operating-level personnel.

Thus, the Commission is recommending that graduate education for public health be structured with academic responsibilities divided among existing institutions according to the functions that their graduates are expected to assume in the field. The schools of public health would concentrate on specialty training of biostatisticians and epidemiologists, and on the training of research scientists, educators, and those preparing for executive and leadership functions after graduation. Training of operating specialty personnel will be primarily at the various other graduate schools of the university. Advanced doctoral training will undoubtedly be concentrated in the schools of public health for most of these specialties, although some schools of engineering are capable of providing doctoral education in certain aspects of environmental health. Similarly, some schools of public administration confer a doctorate with a concentration in health administration.

Functions of Baccalaureate Programs

The baccalaureate preparation for public health is still a relatively small endeavor, and there is little evidence upon which to base strong conclusions as to its desirability. The Commission feels, however, that there is no reason to believe that baccalaureate programs are incapable of providing a small proportion of trained entry-level personnel who can at least be expected to perform more adequately than persons with no training whatsoever.

Meeting Other Needs

These categories are not mutually exclusive. It is probable that some people may start their careers in public health as one type of professional and will later move on to positions with broader functions. Thus, some clinical specialists or some public health nurses, for example, may originally function in a narrow, restricted role. Later they may demonstrate such ability and interest as to suggest they are qualified for policy-making, executive activity. We believe that it would be desirable for such people to return for midcareer training in a school of public health so that they can be exposed to the complete range of the knowledge base at such time as their responsibilities and functions demand a comprehensive overview of the whole field of public health. Until that time, their educational needs might not require the range of resources best provided in schools of public health.

There are undoubtedly other ways in which higher education for public health for a group of disparate professional functions could be restructured. These might involve establishing new forms of education and new academic institutions. We believe that the urgent need for change dictates the use of existing resources in the most expedient manner possible. Within the framework we will outline there are alternative ways to achieve the desired results, but the different schools and programs providing higher education for public health will have to devise the precise means within the limitations of their own goals and resources. We hope to initiate a process of specific goal delineation by setting out a set of principles for the education of public health professionals and leadership. It remains for those directly concerned with these important endeavors to evaluate and implement these principles in their own way.

Recommendation

4. *There should be a major redirection and reorganization of higher education for public health, based on the recognition that different groups of personnel with different functions will require different kinds of educational programs.*

A. *The schools of public health should concentrate their efforts primarily on:*

    (1) *The preparation of people who will function as executives, planners, and policy-makers.*

    (2) *The preparation of epidemiologists and biostatisticians.*

    (3) *The preparation of research scientists and educators.*

B. *Individual graduate programs in other schools in universities should continue concentrating on the preparation of people who who will function at the operating level in respective specialty fields of public health.*

8. The Schools
of Public Health

Like other academic institutions in recent years, many schools of public health have been involved in a systematic process of self-study, re-examining their goals and objectives and the means for achieving them. The results of these efforts are not yet apparent in the form of major changes in the schools' functions or reputations. In fact, the schools of public health have all been criticized both by graduates of the schools and by people in the field. The Commission has heard from several sources comments such as: "The schools of public health are dead; the only thing left for the Commission to do is to bury them."

It is true that, for some schools, there are people inside as well as outside who question whether the schools have outlived their usefulness as separate academic entities in the university, and there are questions about the quality and relevance of the educational programs in all the schools. But the Commission believes that there is a potential for excellence in the schools of public health which could have value for all public health education and which should be nurtured.

Statement of Intent

As a group, the schools of public health now educate the complete range of graduate degree-holding personnel for public health. In addition to giving doctoral training in special fields, they undertake to train for executive functions while simultaneously training first level professionals in specialty service areas. This approach has been defended on the grounds that the educational process toward leadership involves a continuum of experience which must not be broken by apportioning different parts of it to different educational institutions, or else a new problem of educational fragmentation will be created. However, this "fragmentation" is a fact today, as more and more first level professionals are receiving their training outside schools of public health. In view of this, the Commission believes it would be wiser to give purposeful structure to this division of educational responsibility, rather than to continue unplanned efforts which, in effect, result in competition for those students preparing to be first level professionals while neglecting the important group of leadership personnel now conspicuous by their absence in the field.

Many schools claim that they are able to educate for leadership in public health as well as prepare operating level personnel by providing different educational tracks for students with different backgrounds. In health administration, for example, nine schools have differentiated programs for students with professional backgrounds and for those with no experience in public health or a related discipline. Health professionals are eligible for the M.P.H. degree, while all others receive either a variation of the master's degree (M.S., M.S.P.H., M.S. Hyg., etc.) or enroll in an expanded and longer M.P.H. program. Even in these schools, however, all students usually share the same introductory courses and take many of the same courses in health administration regardless of their level of preparation. Seven schools do not appear to have differentiated tracks at all. These conditions also obtain in the mix of students in other fields. This creates dissatisfaction and serious problems for students and faculty which outweigh the theoretical advantages of socializing students with greatly varied backgrounds in the same basic courses. Special exercises designed to achieve this integrative purpose hold greater promise and are not likely to have the inherent disadvantages described above. At present, the separate tracks for students with different backgrounds are not sufficiently differentiated.

While it is possible for education for operating-level and leadership personnel to take place under the same roof, the Commission believes that it may be essentially dysfunctional. It is palpably detrimental to education if students with sophisticated knowledge must sit in classes where time is inevitably spent explaining material familiar to some and a mystery to others. While it has been stated that teaching hospitals simultaneously train young physicians as well as nurses, we view this situation as quite different from the one existing in a school of public health. Responsibility for physician education rests with a different authority from that for nurses, and the faculty, curriculum, as well as academic hours are for the most part totally separate. A closer analogy might be found in a dental school, but even here the program for dental hygienists does not overlap with that for dental students. Surely, a business school would never merge the educational program for corporate vice-presidents with the program for recent college graduates?

We believe that one way in which the schools of public health could meet some of the mounting criticism which has been directed at them in recent years would be for them to elect to function more effectively at advanced graduate levels. They could then concentrate on the substantial job for which they are uniquely suited, namely to provide doctoral training in specialty areas, to prepare biostatisticians and epidemiologists, to expand research and knowledge in public health, and to educate people for executive functions in public health. This means that schools of public health would have to reduce their current programs for training subspecialists, such as health educators, hospital administrators, and public health nurses, unless these specialists were returning to school for advanced training for executive functions in their specialty. If this change in mission is adopted, the schools will naturally have to make changes both in their admission criteria and in their educational programs.

Any substantial change in policy in most of the schools would be expected to take time and to result in some temporary dislocation. Nevertheless, implementation must begin with a recognition of the need for change and a commitment by each school to a new policy of educational selectivity. Whatever decision an individual school makes about its perception of its role should be articulated so that the university administration is clearly informed of what it can expect from its school of public health. If the Commission's recommendation is adopted, some current responsibilities will be dropped by the school of public health and will perhaps be placed in other graduate programs within the same university. Some may be carried out in cooperation with other institutions while still others may be discarded completely. Decisions will have to be made that are consistent not only with the total situation in a particular university but also in the context of regional needs and resources. Some schools may be in a stage of development which would preclude implementation of such a plan in the near future. A clearly articulated statement should still be prepared by each school of public health in terms of its commitment to the education of a defined and limited group of students, its plan for implementation of this policy, and its proposals for educating the different groups of students now served during the interim period before any new policy is totally implemented. This statement, naturally, should be reviewed and approved by the university administration, who will have to assume responsibility for any indicated relocation of educational programs.

Recommendation

5. Each school of public health should develop a clear statement of its educational mission and the plan that it has developed for the preparation of personnel for executive and leadership roles in public health in general, and in the specialties of public health practice, the training of epidemiologists, biostatisticians, research scientists, and educators. This statement must have the concurrence and support of the university administration.

Schools of Public Health as Regional Resources

We recognize that this suggestion of a clearly defined role for the schools of public health runs counter to certain recent trends. In the past few years several state legislatures have established schools of public health at their state universities for the sole expressed purpose of providing manpower for state public health programs. It is unlikely that either the schools or these government bodies will take kindly to the suggestion that the schools now concentrate on the education of a smaller group of students and ignore the needs for staff public health nurses, health and hospital administrators, or health educators. However, the other models we have described can train much of this needed manpower less expensively than can the schools of public health, as they should be able to make use of existing course offerings and faculty on a shared basis. They do not have to recruit full-time faculty for limited, although important, activities. Programs in other graduate schools are designed primarily, if not expressly, to educate the entry level professionals in certain fields to meet the day-to-day demands of ongoing programs. If the new role for the schools of public health is viewed as developing in tandem with a clearly recognized role for other educational efforts in public health, it is clear that a cooperative unification of the total effort could be achieved.

This would mean that the schools of public health would have to function as regional resources which would be consulted about, and would participate in, academic planning for other graduate programs in higher education for public health within specified geographic areas. These schools possess the faculty and other resources in the central elements of the knowledge base, as well as active programs in environmental health, which should be used to nourish all education for public health. Their contribution can be maximized at least cost if the schools themselves seed teaching programs throughout a region, instead of attempting to collect all students from that region on their own premises.

As an academic resource, the school would address itself to the educational needs for public health in an entire region. Its faculty would be available to assist faculties in medical and other health-related schools in other universities to develop teaching programs and plan research in public health. Furthermore, as a service resource the school would provide consultation services—for example, to communities and states in the region for the development and evaluation of field programs.

There are enough public health schools in all regions of the United States for their influence to be spread profitably over all areas of the nation. Table 3 and Figure 1 show the present location of schools of public health in the United States by geographic region. Table 4 indicates the residence of graduates of schools of public health by region in 1970 (White et al., 1974).

Table 3

Schools of Public Health by Regions

Regions	State Schools	Private Schools	Total Number	1970 Pop. (millions)	Population per School (millions)
New England	Massachusetts	Harvard, Yale	3	11.75	3.92
Middle Atlantic	—	Pittsburgh, Columbia	2	37.12	18.56
East North Central	Illinois, Michigan	—	2	40.21	20.11
West North Central	Minnesota	—	1	16.29	16.29
South Atlantic	North Carolina, South Carolina	Hopkins	3	30.72	10.24
East South Central	—	—	0	12.78	—
West South Central	Oklahoma, Texas	Tulane	3	19.38	6.46
Mountain	—	—	0	8.25	—
Pacific	Washington, California, Berkeley, Los Angeles, Hawaii	Loma Linda	5	26.60	5.32
Puerto Rico	Puerto Rico	—	1	3.09	3.09
Totals	13	7	20	206.20	10.31

Source: White et al., A Survey of 1956–1972 Graduates of American Schools of Public Health. Bureau of Manpower Education Contract NIH 71-459. The Johns Hopkins University, December 1974.

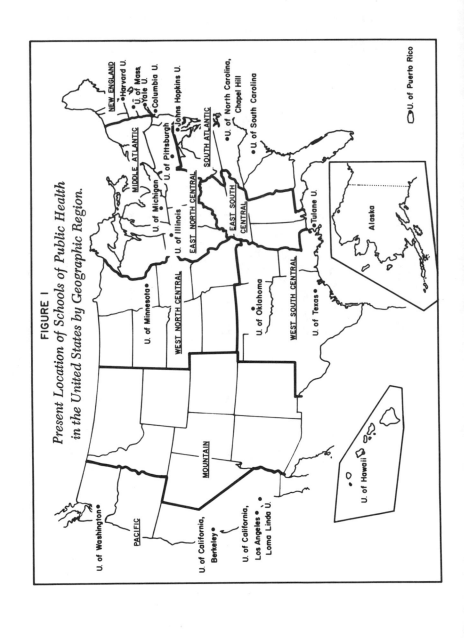

FIGURE I

Present Location of Schools of Public Health in the United States by Geographic Region.

Table 4

**Geographic Division of Residence of Graduates
Compared to the Population of the United States in 1970**

Geographic Division of Residence in the U.S. Pop.	Percent Total Graduates at Time of Survey[2]	Total Population 1970[3]	Ratio of Percent of Graduates to Percent of Total Pop.
New England	6.9	5.7	1.21
Middle Atlantic	16.1	18.0	.89
East North Central	12.5	19.5	.64
West North Central	4.0	7.9	.50
South Atlantic	19.8	14.9	1.33
East South Central	3.3	6.2	.53
West South Central	6.9	9.4	.73
Mountain	5.2	4.0	1.30
Pacific	19.8	12.9	1.53
Puerto Rico and outlying areas of U.S.[1]	5.5	1.5	3.66
Total	100.0	100.0	

[1] Includes Guam, Virgin Islands of the U.S., American Samoa, Midway, Wake Island, the Canal Zone, and Trust Territory of the Pacific Islands.

[2] Excludes graduates living in foreign countries and those not reporting place of residence.

[3] Excludes U.S. population living outside the 50 states and the District of Columbia, Puerto Rico, and outlying areas; and federal employees, including armed forces and their dependents, crews on merchant ships, and other citizens.

Source: White et al., "A Survey of 1956–1972 Graduates of American Schools of Public Health." Bureau of Manpower Education Contract NIH 71-459. The Johns Hopkins University, December 1974.

In several schools of public health a substantial portion of the student body now comes from out-of-state, but from within the region served by the school. For example, 20 percent of Tulane's students come from southern states other than Louisiana, and 11 percent of the University of Minnesota's students come from other West North Central states.

Other schools of public health act as service resources for their state or region. At the University of Washington, the Department of Health Services participates in a Health Policy Analysis Program, designed to provide nonbiased research and analysis services to the public decision makers in the state who are responsible for health care issues and policies. The school also conducted a Technical Assistance and Continuing Education project which provided services to state and local health planning agencies in Washington, Oregon, Alaska, and Idaho.

Columbia University School of Public Health in New York City currently has a contract with New York State Department of Social Services to train their staff for the statewide Medicaid program. For some time the School has provided continuing education for the senior administrative personnel of the New York State Department of Mental Hygiene. Columbia's program of continuing education has a long-standing arrangement with the Health Department of the neighboring state of New Jersey to provide educational programs for their staff, particularly health officers. Columbia's School of Public Health has also assisted several New Jersey institutions and agencies in their health-related programs. Newark College of Arts and Sciences of Rutgers University is interested in establishing a baccalaureate program in public health, and Columbia has advised them on that process, has agreed to collaborate in training programs, and is currently in the process of training faculty. Columbia has also advised the New Jersey Department of Higher Education, Office of Health Professions Education, which requested assistance in developing guidelines for the training of specialists and generalists in public health, as part of the State's Health Professions Education Master Plan.

The University of Michigan's School of Public Health is working with the state's four medical schools, the State Office of Health Planning, the regional health planning agencies, and the Michigan Association of Regional Medical Programs to establish a health planning technical assistance center based in the School of Public Health, to provide technical assistance to Michigan's health planning agencies. The School's Community Blood Pressure Control Project and an internal faculty-student task force are providing technical assistance through the City of Detroit Health Department for a systematic blood pressure control program for Detroit residents. In Detroit, the School is participating in a two-university consortium designed to provide advisory services through the City Planning Department on a variety of problems.

Although regulations vary from state to state and can serve as impediments to free-flowing exchange of knowledge, students, and faculty, existing regional compacts demonstrate that it is possible to surmount the obstacles. Other examples of regional cooperation already exist in the field of higher education. The Western

Interstate Commission for Higher Education, financed in large part by the 13 participating western states, was formed in 1951 to assist colleges, universities, and students, and to expedite the expansion of a supply of specialized manpower in the west on an organized cooperative basis. For example, student exchange programs at co-operating schools provide opportunities for professional education when a given specialty is not offered within the boundaries of the sending state, and may involve interstate exchange of money (Western Interstate Commission for Higher Education, 1972).

The Southern Regional Education Board, representing 14 south-ern states, has developed an "academic common market," through which each member state puts a number of its unique educational programs in a "market pool" and then arranges for its residents to have access on a resident-tuition basis to those out-of-state programs not offered at its own institutions. This program is being expanded to try to include private as well as public universities. Other pro-grams provide for sharing of scarce or expensive academic installa-tions such as an electron microscope, wind tunnel, or nuclear reactor (Southern Regional Educational Board, 1974).

Under a contract with the SREB, the School of Public Health at the University of North Carolina reserves places for students from Kentucky and West Virginia. These students are considered as in-state and pay tuition as if they came from North Carolina. The SREB pays the difference to the University and collects from the states of Kentucky and West Virginia.

While the frameworks of these compacts are not necessarily the ones that would be appropriate for all schools of public health to copy, they give some idea of the mechanisms that could be used.

Financial Support

If a school of public health is to act as a regional resource it will have to embark upon such a course deliberately. This will involve establishing liaison with other schools and universities in the region using whatever auspices are available. It will also mean developing plans in conjunction with official government agencies. It would not be possible for a school of public health to act as a regional resource without financial assistance for this specific purpose, and federal and state governments are the logical source of such assistance. As we have emphasized before, the cost of such funding to a state government, for example, would be far less than the cost of establishing an independent full scale school of public health.

The Commission does not intend to suggest that the schools of public health impose their expertise on other institutions. But the possibilities for cooperative arrangements which will utilize the resources of the schools to the optimum capacity should be explored. And if the schools of public health do not initiate such explorations, who will?

Recommendations

6. *The schools of public health should provide technical assistance for the growing number of programs in other parts of the university which train certain types of manpower for the field. They should serve as regional resources to consult and participate in academic planning with all graduate programs in higher education for public health within specified geographic areas.*

7. *Federal and state governments should provide financial support which will enable and encourage schools of public health to fulfill important functions as regional resources for the production of appropriately trained manpower for public health.*

Admission Requirements

Until the 1960s or thereabouts, the student body in schools of public health consisted chiefly of individuals who already had degrees in a profession such as medicine, dentistry, or engineering. Many of these also had experience in public health activity. During the past decade, however, the schools have been accepting younger students straight out of college, and there are now many more entrants with neither experience nor a professional degree. This policy has been defended on the grounds that, until the schools began admitting young students fresh from a baccalaureate degree, public health as a field was unable to attract the best young minds to work in it. Poor civil service pay scales and unstimulating work environments have been blamed for the inability of public health agencies to compete for bright young people. But many young doctors, lawyers, and other professionals choose to work in poverty programs, the Peace Corps, or other relatively low-paying service programs with an idealistic purpose. Therefore, we do not believe that pay scales are the deciding factor for the "best young minds." It is more probable that the low profile of public health activity is responsible for the observed unpopularity of public health agencies. Today there are other pathways—via the graduate programs in other schools of the university—which provide an entry into professional public health activity for the bright young college graduate.

Whatever the merits of the arguments on either side of this question, the desirability of admitting people fresh from college into a school of public health depends upon the mission of each school. If, as the Commission has recommended, the schools of public health concentrate on specific limited goals, then there will be very little purpose served by admitting people with no graduate degrees, except in biostatistics and epidemiology. Mathematics or statistics majors are probably ready to specialize in biostatistics immediately after graduating from college. However, college graduates who elect epidemiology as a career are likely to be ill-equipped for the course of study in a school of public health unless they have had a fair amount of field experience in epidemiology or have acquired a relevant graduate or professional degree first. In fact, some epidemiology departments which admit young baccalaureates to their programs in schools of public health have required a longer period of time for study and have had to provide compensatory courses in basic medical sciences for such students. Nevertheless, it is possible for such departments to make up for their students' lack of training and experience if they so desire, and still turn out adequate first-level epidemiologists. However, it is impossible to conceive of students fresh from college as appropriate candidates for the group who are expected to perform executive functions in the field.

Therefore, the Commission is also recommending that the schools change their admission requirements. In 1942, the Committee on Professional Education of the American Public Health Association developed a recommendation which said that, ". . . special professional training in public health is best obtained at a well-equipped teaching institution. Such training should be at the graduate level, that is, after earning the professional degree" (Committee on Professional Education, 1942:1533). We believe that this recommendation, with modification, still applies in regard to students who are being prepared for executive and leadership positions. It is obvious that if the schools of public health accept responsibility for the mission the Commission has recommended, there will be very few students fresh from college that the schools themselves will want to admit.

Although the American Public Health Association Committee referred only to professional degrees, this Commission believes that a graduate degree in a field relevant to public health is usually an excellent preparation for the education to be provided by a school of public health. People who have graduate degrees in one of the biologic sciences, or in sociology or economics, possess a substantial amount of relevant background information related to the knowledge base, and this is true, too, for those with field experience in a public health program. For many years it has been widely recognized that experience provides a familiarity with the field which is a reasonably adequate substitute for prior degrees in that it acquaints one with the language and methods of public health.

Changing the admission requirements at the schools will not, of itself, eliminate some of the curricular problems posed by a diverse student body with prior degrees from many professional fields. Lawyers and engineers may well lack the knowledge of normal physiology and disease processes necessary for adequate understanding of the nature and rationale of patient care standards or the health effects of environmental hazards. Similarly, physicians or dentists are probably not sufficiently prepared in the social sciences to understand properly the public policy process or such matters as changing group definitions of health and disease. Schools of public health should either set admission standards in relation to these broad areas of knowledge or should be sure that necessary compensatory courses are provided early in the student's program and as prerequisites for other courses.

Recommendation

8. Schools of public health should require that before admission to their program of training for executive and leadership functions students have either:

    (1) A professional degree in one of the health professions.
    (2) A graduate degree in a field relevant to public health.
    (3) A minimum of three years' experience in a public health program.

Entering students should have an adequate knowledge of the biologic basis of health problems and the basic concepts of social and behavioral sciences so that they can understand the background of the economic, social and political aspects of public health, or schools should plan for, and ensure that, necessary compensatory courses are provided early in the student's educational program.

Organization of Public Health School Faculty

The administrative organization of schools of public health reflects the complexity of educational needs. Whether the structural components of a school be departments, divisions, or program subunits, they include a mixture of disciplines in both the faculty and the student body. The schools of public health with large student bodies are characterized by a large number of individual departments or divisions.

In one such school there are at least five autonomous departments with joint interests, and overlapping and interdependent responsibilities. Health administration is the basic substrate that is fundamental to these departments, yet these departments function autonomously. They develop courses for their own students with their own faculty, rather than sharing important areas of interest and competence, such as concepts and methods, planning, evaluation, the assessment and measurement of health status, and principles of organization and management. Except for crosslisting a few courses which are taken by students from any of the five departments, there is very little interaction between the departments. At the faculty level there is a significant absence of joint delineation of problems or joint development of research activities and curricula.

With the increase of categorically-oriented public health programs in the United States there has followed an increase of categorically-oriented teaching programs. In recent decades there has been increasing specialization, even at the master's level, as compared with earlier periods when training was of a more general character. Special divisions or departments of maternal and child health have been followed by the establishment of specialty programs in mental health, chronic disease, accident control, and the care of long-term illness, among others. All provide their students with instruction in program planning and administration, which is or can be provided in departments of health services administration, and with instruction in research methods and evaluation, which can be provided by the departments of statistics and epidemiology. There is little need for autonomous departments or divisions to organize programs for specialists in these fields. A basic program in health administration, with groupings of added courses in various specialities, would not only be more economic but would also provide superior education.

For example, six schools of public health have designated faculty for special programs of study in public health nursing. Some nurses at schools of public health enroll in the department of public health nursing, while other nurses in the same school study general administration, both preparing for executive positions in public health nursing. The Commission believes that enrollment of nurses in the health administration program will be the more effective for leadership purposes. The specialty program often duplicates courses, which precludes optimum utilization of available resources in other departments. This problem is particularly acute in the teaching of such subjects as planning, evaluation, research methods, and administration.

The field of maternal and child health (MCH) provides a classic example of categorical orientation to the provision of services and, in turn, the organization of professional education.

During the 1960s MCH services were greatly expanded through the provision of federal project grants for comprehensive maternity and infant care, programs for children and youth centers, children's dental health, family planning, and neonatal intensive care. At the same time, special projects, training grants, and teaching and research programs in MCH received increased federal support in the form of grants for these related academic purposes. In 1963 only 30 graduate degrees were awarded to students majoring in MCH teaching programs in schools of public health. A survey of 11 schools conducted in 1973 indicated that the number of MCH degree candidates had increased to over 300 (White, 1973).

The average MCH teaching program now has at least nine faculty members of diverse academic and professional backgrounds. These may include physicians, nurses, nutritionists, biostatisticians, child development experts, mental health professionals, health planners, medical care administrators, and behavioral scientists. The subject matter of courses offered by MCH programs has also been expanded. The traditional concentration on such topics as the operation of child health and maternity services or the epidemiology of disease processes has been supplemented by such areas as nutrition, human sexuality, family planning, demography, management and administration, and child development.

The curriculum for MCH students now varies considerably from one school to another. Although many schools retain the concept of a core curriculum, differing emphases are placed on biostatistics, epidemiology, the biologic and social sciences, and public health practice. As the number of MCH courses has grown, there has been a tendency to design clusters of courses around areas of interest such as family planning, family life, planning and administration, and health assessment. Emphasis is now placed on courses dealing with the planning, organization, administration, and research methodology for the evaluation of health services for mothers and children in a variety of settings. Approximately half a dozen programs have explicitly defined objectives for training the nonmedical administrator.

Within the schools of public health there are various organizational structures for the teaching of MCH. Some schools have large departments, others have relatively independent programs within departments such as health administration, while still others may have faculty members in this specialty but no administratively separated program. Some programs place heavy reliance on courses taught jointly with other units, and some have enrolled students in joint teaching programs with other schools in the university.

Recently there has been a great increase in the number and variety of professional and other groups which express interest in promoting the optimal health and development of children. Different schools in the university have departments of pediatrics, pediatric nursing, child psychiatry, special education, and many others. Similarly, in the community there has been a proliferation of voluntary agencies, parents' groups, and children's lobbies actively furthering the cause of the health and welfare of children.

Citizens and agencies concerned with the health of mothers and children no longer have a single clear focus for the expression of their concerns. The current trend toward the development of systems of personal health services to serve entire populations regardless of age or categorical health needs complicates the problem. At the same time, new special purpose programs for early childhood and adolescence have tended to develop independently of the traditional services for mothers and children.

The special teaching activities dilute the role of MCH teaching programs. Their objectives and curricula now overlap those of many other academic programs. Within the university, as well as in society at large, there is little effective coordination of the many efforts for child health. This problem is also seen in the confused variety of federal and state agencies responsible for health, welfare, and educational services to children and family units.

No spokesman for reorganization of public health education would propose the deletion of a focus on the special needs of mothers and children. In service programs there is an obvious need for general skills in planning, administration, management and program evaluation, but the effectiveness of these services also requires the skills of professionals with interest and competency in child health and development. However, the competency of professionals in MCH does not depend upon administratively-independent MCH teaching programs. A variety of administrative structures is now used to present MCH teaching, and there is no evidence that graduates of autonomous MCH departments are more competent than MCH professionals who were not educated in administratively separate programs.

The principles illustrated by the teaching of MCH apply equally to other categorical programs, among which are public health nursing, mental health, and hospital administration. In these and other areas there are autonomous departments and divisions which unnecessarily duplicate and compete for resources.

One problem that schools of public health encounter, as do other schools, stems from the important tradition of autonomy. The autonomy and academic freedom of the individual faculty member protect faculty views and opinions, and do not free them from the responsibility of presenting those views in coordination with a planned departmental program related to subject matter. The faculty member should not function autonomously in relation to other faculty in his specialty.

The tradition of individual faculty freedom is often translated operationally into a concept of autonomy for a department itself. This independence properly encourages the department to develop its own initiatives and to recruit staff which can contribute as directly as possible to the mission of the department. However, autonomy can, and often does, result in isolation from other departments.

If the degree of isolation is sufficiently great, one result is that the department will duplicate work being done in other departments of the school. The same department may also ignore those opportunities and needs perceived in other parts of the school as ones which should be met by that department. In addition, departmental autonomy has, in several notable instances, increased the isolation of the entire school from other relevant academic resources in the university, by building faculty resources in one department when these are already represented on campus as the university's major investment in the discipline.

Without sacrificing the important principle of academic freedom, schools of public health can, and would be wise to, modify their departmental structure in such a way as to have fewer departments, with effective continuous communication between departments, other units in the university, and the field of practice.

Recommendation

9. In order to overcome the isolation of faculty compartmentalization, the faculty of schools of public health should be organized so that related skills and knowledge will be unified for teaching and research.

Avoidance of Unnecessary Duplication of Faculty

Education for public health has not had adequate input from the social sciences, particularly from such fields as economics, sociology, and the management sciences. Special consideration needs to be given to the optimal manner of integrating social science research and teaching into schools of public health. Most schools have incorporated social science faculty into various departments, such as epidemiology or health administration. A few schools have set up distinct departments in the social sciences.

The Commission believes that it is unwise to set up departments in a school of public health when these fields are already effectively represented elsewhere in the university. Social sciences can best be taught through cooperative arrangements with such departments as economics, sociology, and psychology. It is reasonable to expect that these departments would consistently represent a high level of knowledge and research in these fields. Though such departments do not always adapt their disciplines readily to other fields, the effort and time spent on developing appropriate arrangements can be justified by the expectation that effective two-way interchange between these basic social science departments and schools of public health will result in benefits to each.

Similarly, in the biomedical sciences, cooperative arrangements would be of value. A few schools of public health have strong and effective activities in certain biomedical fields such as virology and parasitology. These are disciplines cognate to public health which are needed and consistently found in schools of medicine. Questions can be asked about the long-term validity of locating them in a school of public health. This is not to say that these fields do not have pertinence to the training of selected professionals in public health, but often this could be arranged more effectively and economically through a cooperative interchange with a medical school.

Schools of public health often claim that they are forced to develop their own resources either because corresponding departments in the university are inadequate, or because these departments show little or no inclination to apply their efforts to problems of public health. When this is the case, a school may indeed have no alternative but to proceed on its own, and the resulting duplication of resources may not only be necessary but may even lead at times to productive interaction within the university. However, the caliber of faculty from a basic discipline to be found in a minidepartment of a school of public health is generally not likely to be as high as that associated with the major center for that discipline in the university.

Schools of public health, like other centers of higher education, must make arrangements for their faculty to conduct scientific research of high quality. This should take into account opportunities within the university as well as in the school so that optimum arrangements for necessary and fruitful collaboration can be developed. However, mere duplication is wasteful and, in the long run, harmful to the quality of education.

Arranging interchange and joint activity among different schools and departments is difficult in any university. However, such arrangements have been successful and could perhaps serve as models for future attempts. For example, the Harvard School of Public Health has developed two M.S. programs which use resources from other schools in the university and from the neighboring Massachusetts Institute of Technology. The two-year curricula in Environmental Management and in Health Policy and Management use existing courses in the John F. Kennedy School of Government, the Graduate School of Arts and Sciences (departments of statistics, economics, and government), the Harvard Business School, the

Graduate School of Design, and the M.I.T. Sloan School of Management. Degrees are awarded by the Harvard School of Public Health.

The Department of Health Administration at the University of North Carolina School of Public Health has different kinds of cooperative arrangements with other university resources. Some health administration students take courses in the School of Business, and faculty time may also be bought to have Business School faculty teach courses in the School of Public Health. As an outgrowth of a five-year joint program with the Department of City and Regional Planning, the School of Public Health maintains joint faculty appointments and co-listing of courses with this department.

There is a compelling logic to establishing cooperative intra-university arrangements. If they are carefully worked through to minimize the natural reluctance of each department or school to give sufficient emphasis to the special interests of other departments and schools, then education and research of higher quality can be expected. In addition to the improvement in quality which can be expected from such arrangements, the more efficient use of resources represents a needed measure in the present period of financial constraints which universities face.

Recommendation

10. In order to ensure high quality and to avoid unnecessary duplication of faculty, the university administration should support and facilitate intrauniversity arrangements which would enable departments in the social, management, and biomedical sciences to work together with faculty in schools of public health wherever this will contribute effectively to meeting the education and research needs of the school.

Funding

The availability of federal funds for special training programs has often led the schools of public health to develop programs in response to funding patterns rather than in relation to a school's more generic educational role. This has resulted in many highly specialized and categorical programs which were developed with a small number of fulltime faculty members and with few criteria, if any, for evaluating the academic effort. When new programs are proposed, either in response to new emphases in health service programs or to new sources of funding, there is a temptation to put such programs into operation even when the optimal facilities or faculty are not available, on the theory that some education is better than none. Many schools have not resisted this temptation, and some of the programs consequently are weak.

Before any new program is instituted it would be wise for decisions to be made about the amount and quality of the effort needed and the minimum number of students desired in that program to make it a valid academic proposition. In doing so, the question of effective use of resources must be faced. If the schools of public health are to concentrate on providing leadership for the field, they will each have to resist the temptation to develop special programs in every new area, no matter how important that area seems to be or how easy it may be to get funding for it.

The granting agency has responsibilities here, too. When special projects are funded to meet specific national needs, these grants should be clearly targeted and time-limited in relation to those needs. This would help to prevent the creation of ongoing programs which do not contribute to the overall mission of the school. The grants should, of course, be awarded competitively on the basis of the adequacy of existing resources.

Recommendation

11. Project grants to meet national needs for specific kinds of public health manpower should be targeted and time-limited for those purposes so that they do not encourage the unnecessary development of permanent programs. Schools should adapt to these short-term needs where they can without altering their long-term objectives.

Centers of Excellence

In recent years schools of public health have emphasized doctoral training programs. In 1974, the 19 schools in operation awarded 197 doctoral degrees (personal communication with W. B. Parsons, 1975). At most of the schools doctorates constituted about 10 percent of the total degrees awarded, five schools awarded no doctoral degrees, and at one school, Johns Hopkins, 20 percent of the total degrees were doctoral degrees.

More than three-quarters of the total number of doctoral degrees are obtained in the four areas of epidemiology, biostatistics, public health administration, and environmental health. However, a small number of doctoral candidates is found in many of the other specialty fields, such as health education, mental health, and nutrition (White et al. 1974).

Most schools of public health have developed specialized interest areas in which they excel, or aim to do so. These can and should serve as centers for doctoral and postdoctoral training for students throughout the country. It is generally recognized, for example, that today the biostatistics department at the University of North Carolina has one of the most advanced programs in the nation. The same distinction is readily accorded to the department of epidemiology at Johns Hopkins. While biostatistics and epidemiology are central to public health, and all schools must represent them in the curriculum, good training at the master's level requires far fewer resources and faculty per student than does training at the doctoral level.

There are other examples of doctoral programs which are not provided at all schools and do not need to be. At least one excellent department of public health nutrition now exists, at Harvard University. In addition, the nutrition department at the University of California at Berkeley, though not in the school of public health, is excellent and provides a good basis for public health nutrition teaching. While we would not presume to prescribe the number of advanced research and training centers in nutrition, we are sure that all schools are not adequately prepared to mobilize the resources necessary for an effective effort at the doctoral level. This is not to gainsay the importance of the subject, as it should be part of the curriculum in all schools of public health.

Similarly with environmental health, where many cognate disciplines contribute to the subject. In fact, much work is now being done outside the schools of public health, in engineering and medical schools, among others. But many problems in environmental health require the special contributions of biostatistics and epidemiology to identify hazards and their effects on human health, and to evaluate control measures. Environmental health is an essential component of public health education, but again we find that not all schools of public health can focus the attention and resources on this subject that are required for doctoral training.

There are other specialties in the field of public health which deserve at least one center for advanced training, but not one in every school. For example, the School of Public Health at the University of Minnesota offers an extensive program in the specifically veterinary aspects of public health in conjunction with the College of Veterinary Medicine. One such program in the nation is probably sufficient, although all schools of public health should continue to provide generalist education to graduate veterinarians who elect such training.

It is obvious that the excellent advanced programs that exist today did not emerge full grown in their first years and the Commission does not mean to suggest curtailing the development of new doctoral programs in the schools of public health. If a school is prepared to make the investment and has the necessary faculty and other resources needed for a good doctoral program, such a program might well fill a demonstrable need. But the natural tendency of those in charge of academic programs and institutions to encourage aggrandizement of educational programs should be resisted. Schools of public health which do not possess distinctive or even adequate resources in a specialized field would be well advised to resist the temptation to compete in such areas at an advanced level; the resulting programs are not likely to serve the students well.

In an economy of scarcity it is important that questions of quality, need, and efficiency be evaluated carefully and objectively in relation to doctoral and postdoctoral programs, particularly before new programs are instituted. Indeed, where only small numbers of doctoral candidates are now being trained in a department, a school would do well to examine the validity of continuing such advanced training.

The Commission wishes to emphasize that it is not trying to discourage the natural and appropriate growth of new areas of strength and advanced specialization within a school. However, every department in every school does not have to strive to develop doctoral programs at the earliest possible date. Each school should undertake, with outside experts, to evaluate its own strengths and weaknesses to determine where such programs might best be encouraged. Strong departments in other schools should be recognized and acknowledged as centers for advanced training and research. These centers could then serve as foci for special professional programs, attracting students from all over the country and assisting other schools of public health and selected educational programs.

Recommendation

12. To protect and support high standards, and to avoid costly competition and duplication of resources, all schools of public health should recognize that certain schools have particular strengths in specialized areas, and are national centers of excellence. Thus, doctoral training and research in these fields should be concentrated at these centers.

The Importance
of Field Experience

Most educational programs for public health are designed to prepare professionals for practice in the field. The problem is deciding how to achieve a balance between the immediate, perceived needs of the field and the more theoretical and long-range approach developed in academia. Both are important. Currently much public health education is considered to be too theoretical by directors of field agencies, who criticize graduates as inadequately prepared to meet the realities of the field.

There are two ways in which this valid criticism can be met, and both should be implemented concurrently. First, the exposure of both students and faculty to the impact of field experience should be increased, and second, field agencies and organizations should have more influence on the curriculum itself.

Just as in education for the practice of medicine, basic science and clinical experience are inseparable, so are the basic sciences and field experience inseparable in education for public health. Teaching and field experience in public health were originally congruent. In fact, the practitioners were the teachers, as they had been in medicine. It is only in recent decades that teaching and the preparation for it have become careers in themselves.

As the science of public health has grown, the search for knowledge as an end in itself has come to preoccupy an increasing proportion of the faculty, who assume that this will of itself assure improvement in the quality of educational programs. In the process, the relationship with field activity has been sacrificed. With few exceptions, field experience is looked at merely as a way to relate the reality of the field to the more important theory of the classroom, and is provided largely to give students a bird's eye view of the day-to-day realities of professional practice. This controverts the growing conviction of some academicians and virtually all practitioners that, although the need for field experience in public health may vary with the individual student and the area of specialization, faculty, students, and participating agencies can all benefit from a closer relationship.

Much of the inadequacy of field experience for students lies in the indirect, episodic, and nonoperational involvement of faculty in student field programs. Many faculty members spend more time in field work in foreign countries than they do in the region of the school. They thus have neither the interest in, nor experience with, health problems and organizations in their region and nationally which responsible field supervision requires. The most effective relationship between the classroom and the field depends upon the involvement of students and faculty in responsible, active service which is then integrated into the total educational experience.

Through their field training activities, schools of public health could make a significant contribution to promoting the health of residents of the surrounding community. However, more often than not, the schools do not seek participation in field programs relevant to local health problems. As a result, many students are unable to relate classroom theory to the actualities of public health practice.

Even in such essentially analytic and mathematical disciplines as biostatistics and epidemiology, there is need for an intimate acquaintance with the real world from which data are acquired and to which analyses are presented. Field experience is even more crucial to such areas as program planning and the organization and management of services.

There are several ways of bringing the practice field to the classroom—visiting and adjunct faculty from the field, simulated games, case studies and consultations—and all of these have their own advantages and disadvantages. In their favor is the fact that they offer some elements of real practice without eliminating faculty control over the student's learning situation. Agency clients are protected from being misused in the name of education, and with simulated games, the test process can be slowed down, diagnosed, and repeated if necessary.

The disadvantages, of course, are that correspondence to reality is always questionable. This may not be crucial for an experienced practitioner who can relate simulated experience to what he has already encountered. For the student who has only classroom knowledge of public health skills and procedures, there is no substitute for a natural, uncontrived setting. Therefore, the Commission wishes to emphasize the importance of getting both students and faculty into the field. The most effective relationship between the classroom and the field depends upon the involvement of students and faculty in responsible, active service which is then integrated into the total educational experience.

In the context of the supervised field placement, students can learn by experience to appreciate the pragmatic dimensions of their specialties. For example, through direct personal exposure to the problems of data collection, a biostatistician will learn the limitations and possibilities implicit in the design and execution of certain types of studies crucial to progress in public health. Students who have not had work experience before starting graduate education, or who have had only limited exposure to health-related work environments, will be able to develop and broaden professional attitudes and perspectives, identify with role models, and gain in self-confidence through observations and practice in the field. Work/study opportunities will permit students to apply the knowledge and skills learned in academia within an agency setting and provide valuable exposure to the professional and sociopolitical milieu of their future practice.

Academic learning takes on new meaning in the light of experience in practice, and this experience gives to the student and the faculty new meaning for the academic material. It is the interaction between the two that becomes the real essence of preparation for professional practice and research. This type of experience can also be crucial to the development of effective research on certain problems.

If the touchstone for the students is "work/study," the touchstone for faculty is "work/teach." Both academic institutions and their faculty members benefit from continuing participation in field activities. Combining work and teaching as a faculty responsibility is imperative to vitalize the curriculum, to enliven the teaching/learning activities, and to stimulate and facilitate needed research activities.

Field responsibilities may not be appropriate for all faculty members or in all subjects. However, it is difficult to see how the teaching of health administration, environmental health, and population sciences, for example, can remain relevant unless those involved have a continuous exposure to, and relationship with, the problems of operating agencies.

For a long time the combined roles of teacher and researcher have been accepted as appropriate for all faculty. Yet it is being increasingly recognized that without constant contact with the workplace, teaching becomes stale and too academic. For this reason it is time to think of a work and teaching combination as equally appropriate and necessary for faculty as research and teaching. Both are needed. Those teachers who deal with the basic sciences may need less of a working relationship with the field, as do the preclinical science teachers in the medical schools.

Epidemiologists, biostatisticians and environmental specialists are increasingly employed in health and health-related agencies. There is no reason why some of them cannot combine such activities with some academic responsibilities. This could be accomplished in a number of ways. If the salary scales and fringe benefits are equivalent, it would be possible for one to teach part-time, or for another to work in the field full-time for a few years and then to teach for a few years. Public health education programs in institutions other than public health schools (engineering schools, schools of nursing, schools of public administration, etc.) could impose the same requirements on faculty to work *and* teach, in tandem or in series.

Arrangements and requirements of this nature are increasingly feasible in view of the changes that are taking place in government-supported public health activities. Title IV of the Intergovernmental Personnel Act of 1970 (5 U.S.C. 3371-3376) now authorizes temporary assignment of personnel to work in state and local governments and institutions of higher education (reciprocal arrangements are made but are not necessarily one to one).

The concentration of program responsibility in the Public Health Service and the state health departments is passing to many smaller government units which, in the past, were not staffed or prepared to meet the complex demands now being made upon them. As legislation for consumer protection, environmental protection and national health insurance comes into being, public health responsibilities will inevitably expand. Many of these new activities are now being carried on in various types of organizations without adequately trained professionals. Furthermore, recent legislation which provides for greater consumer participation and local control will in turn require more sophisticated professional training and expertise covering a broader range of subject matter.

Faculty relationships with the field should not merely consist of an occasional consultation or membership on a committee, but should include responsible involvement in a wide range of activities, including the provision of direct and continuous services, even if only on a part-time basis. Faculty should—and in fact a number already do—work with, and for, executive and legislative agencies in all branches of government, as well as with different agencies and groups (unions, voluntary organizations, and others) that exist in the "real world." This bespeaks a new role for the faculty member, not as a visitor and observer, but as a participant, a colleague, even a partner with health agencies and students.

There is also a need for operating agencies to develop a reciprocal relationship with programs of higher education for public health. Agencies should serve as colleagues and collaborators with faculty in planning and supervising the student's experience, and integrating applied and theoretical knowledge, and thus play a major role in shaping the professional perspectives and capabilities of future public health practitioners.

Opportunities should be sought to include the direct and responsible consideration of actual community health problems in formal educational programs. Moreover, by building strong working relationships with public health in educational institutions, agencies can help create a framework for continuous involvement in problem solving and interchange, through which new knowledge and the full range of expertise can be applied directly to field situations

The integration of field study into the public health curriculum on an enlarged and regular basis will create problems which are the inevitable consequences of expanding the academic horizon. One recent study of *Theory in Practice* refers to a series of operational questions which must be answered

> ". . . concerning administrative requirements, credits, supervision, relation to academic coursework, selection of students, definition of student responsibility, and degree of faculty involvement There are, in addition, more serious questions that reflect the mismatch between field experience and the culture of the academy." (Argyris and Schon, 1974)

Field work must be carefully arranged so that it does, in fact, contribute important educational experience. This can be done and the Commission therefore rejects the argument that the period set aside for formal academic instruction should not be tainted with premature vocational emphases.

Opinions concerning the appropriate timing and length of field experience for students and faculty vary, as do attitudes toward the relative value of field experience for students in various specialties of public health, and toward the degree of flexibility appropriate to field programs to meet the needs of individual students. In public health it will also be necessary to determine whether all students must have supervised field experience, regardless of their backgrounds and goals.

Some students and professionals maintain that they gain more from their academic training because they have had previous work experience. If this observation is valid, perhaps academic programs in public health should insist on health-related work experience before admission or upon an acceptable arrangement to provide it during the period of enrollment at the university. Finally, criteria for admission, as well as exemption from field work, must be established; a deliberate and continuous pattern of input from faculty and participating agencies would be of value here.

Other caveats have involved the high cost of appropriate field training to students, faculty, and participating agencies, and the separation of the working student from the scholastic milieu during his period of field service. Cost-benefit ratios in terms of direct financing are difficult to project. But community involvement, faculty commitments of time and expertise, and agency readjustment to absorb student trainees all require detailed examination, and offer promise of minimizing the problems of financing field training. Furthermore, it would be a gross misinterpretation to assume that faculty involvement in the field would represent a cost which is totally additive to present faculty activities. It should be considered as a replacement for at least a significant proportion of the current activities of faculty, providing particularly focused experience in program development, administration, and evaluation.

The Commission believes that while these problems and issues are present to some extent in field programs (or clinical experience) in almost every educational discipline, they are not sufficient justification for the exclusion of practical experience as a major component of higher education for public health. Pejorative connotations often surround the concept of vocational training, particularly in the minds of those who would limit education exclusively to formal academic classroom activity. But an understanding of the practical aspects of the profession as they relate to public health theory would seem to be a necessity for students, and should be acquired before completion of the formal educational program.

Rational discussion of these issues is often impeded because participants fall victim to the tyranny of words. Terms such as "vocational" and "training" are distinguished more sharply than is justifiable from the terms "education" and "academic." These words, of course, are endowed with various meanings by those who use them. Webster's dictionary, however, uses rather similar phrases to define the words "educate" and "train," and it does not seem productive to overemphasize the distinctions between field training and academic education.

Field training typically makes classroom learning more expensive, both in terms of time and of money. However, it is also potentially much more effective. The field experience can and should be organized in such a way that it provides the student with the maximum opportunity to participate in the day-to-day activities and realities of the public health profession, the faculty preceptor with a consistent and rewarding involvement and input into the applied aspects of his academic activity, and the operating agency with a direct contributory relationship.

A restructuring of field study will have benefits for all three groups involved. Students will learn by experience to appreciate the pragmatic dimensions of their specialties. A combination of work and teaching as a faculty responsibility will energize the curriculum, enliven teaching/learning activities, and stimulate and facilitate needed research activities. If a framework for continuous interchange between the school and the field agency is established, new knowledge and the full range of professional expertise can be brought directly to field situations. In short, unless educational institutions preparing professionals for public health develop strong links with health agencies and community organizations, they will serve the public poorly.

Recommendations

13. Supervised programs of field experience in connection with academic activity must be an integral and significant part of education for public health responsibility.

14. Faculty members in schools of public health should undertake periodic, if not continuous, formal responsibilities in the operation of community health services which are relevant to, and will be supportive of, their respective fields of academic responsibility.

15. Educational institutions should develop reciprocal relationships with health agencies and community organizations to bring greater realism to the classroom, and academic expertise to the field. They should also solicit, and be responsive to, evaluations of their educational programs provided by these agencies.

Training of Foreign Nationals

The oldest established schools of public health in the United States have traditionally provided graduate education in public health for students from many foreign countries, who then returned to lead public health activities in their native lands. Foreign students have always been represented in the student bodies of schools of public health. However, during the past decade or more the ratio has declined sharply as American student enrollments have increased. For example, in 1950–51 more than 40 percent of the students registered for the master's degree came from foreign countries (exclusive of Canada). In the 1960s the ratio dropped to 20 percent and by 1970 this ratio decreased further to 17 percent. However, foreign physicians still constitute a substantial portion (40 percent) of the total physician graduates of the schools of public health (Hall et al., 1973b).

In the past it was assumed that the knowledge and skills acquired in the United States by a foreign student would be immediately applicable to the health problems of his native country. While this may have been true to some extent several decades ago, American health problems and the educational emphases of schools preparing public health professionals have altered so radically in recent years that this is no longer the case. Although in varying degrees special seminars and other efforts are made to relate some of the coursework to the less developed regions and nations from which many

Table 5

Summary of Survey of Schools of Public Health
and Schools of Medicine Concerning International Health
(September, 1973)

Questions	Schools of Public Health		Schools of Medicine	
	No. Answering Questions	"Yes"	No. Answering Questions	"Yes"
Have Dept. of Int'l. Health	19	5	62	3
Have Subdivision of Int'l. Health	14	6	59	11
Have Courses in Int'l. Health	18	16	59	18
Have Courses w/ Sections in Int'l Health	17	17	54	27
Offer Credit for Relevant Courses in Other Departments	18	14	51	19
Offer Fieldwork Abroad	19	13	60	38
Have Exchange Program with Foreign School	17	4	54	15
Have Affiliations with Foreign School or Organization	16	7	55	22
Offer Fellowships in Int'l. Health	18	5	49	17
Have Continuing Education in Int'l. Health	18	4	52	5
Have Faculty in Int'l. Health	18	11	56	12
Have Other Faculty with Interests in Int'l. Teaching	18	15	51	26
Have Administrator for Int'l. Health Affairs	19	6	54	23
Recruit Foreign Students	19	6	58	7
Recruit Foreign Students for Int'l. Health Studies	19	7	57	10
Special Counseling for Foreign Students	19	15	56	15
Special Orientation for Foreign Students	19	14	56	14
Have Input by Foreign Students into the Curriculum on Needs of Their Native Countries	18	12	54	12
Have Placement Facilities for Int'l. Health Work or Work Abroad	19	3	53	7
Plan Changes in Int'l Health Programs	18	1	58	7
Have a Specific School Policy Regarding Int'l. Health	16	15	58	29

Source: Report to the Commission by Dr. George Silver.

of the foreign students come, much of the curriculum has become inapplicable to the needs these students will face when they return home.

A survey was conducted by the Commission in 1973 to gather information on the activities of U.S. schools of public health and schools of medicine which train foreign students, and to learn what is being done to train American public health and medical students for public health work abroad and for international health service. Nineteen schools of public health and 62 of the 79 schools of medicine listed by the American Association of Medical Colleges as having a liaison for international affairs completed the questionnaire.

Results indicate a rather thin layer of educational activity in international health. Some attention is paid to international health in almost all the responding schools. (Table 5). However this attention seems rather superficial and elementary, as it consists primarily of survey courses or of reviews of opportunities to work abroad. In only seven schools of public health is epidemiology an integral part of international health education, and in only six schools is there a firm affiliation with an international organization or foreign school that would lend vital substance to the teaching. In the medical schools the teaching of epidemiology is even less evident (19 schools of 79), and affiliation is effective in only 17 schools.

Information obtained from catalogues of public health schools indicates that few schools have depth or range in teaching programs in international health. Some schools of public health have major investments in the international area in family planning and population studies, and in health services organization and planning. These are the areas where foundation and federal support funds have been most abundant. Medical schools have only minimal involvement in teaching in these areas, with slightly less in population studies than in health service administration and organization.

Only seven of the schools of public health make any effort to recruit foreign students, but all schools claim to be interested in foreign students, and almost all provide counseling services to help them circumvent problems of language and acculturation. The largest American university program in international health, at the Johns Hopkins University School of Hygiene and Public Health, offers more than a dozen courses and has more than 50 students enrolled. Half of these are American and half are from foreign countries. Most of the American students have in recent years returned from overseas experience to apply their skills to innovative health-related programs within the United States, such as those in urban ghettoes and in Appalachia.

More and more nations and regions of the world are developing the educational capacity to train their own basic and midlevel manpower for public health activities. The World Health Organization (1973:53) reports that:

"As of 1971 there were approximately 121 schools of public health in the world. They have been mostly established in the present century. If a distinction is made between postgraduate institutions and schools that are primarily undergraduate medical schools offering basic postgraduate public health training, of the 61 schools established in recent years (since 1942) 45 are in the first category and 16 are in the second (i.e., a ratio of almost 3:1)."

Three-quarters of the schools are located in Europe and in North and South America. The balance is distributed unevenly throughout Asia and Africa. Thus it is clear that the role of American schools of public health in training foreign nationals for midlevel public health activities has diminished since 1942 and is no longer of major importance. It will undoubtedly continue to diminish as other countries develop educational programs more attuned to meeting their specific national needs.

However, there remains a need for American schools to provide education at more advanced levels for service, research, and academic training in such fields as epidemiology, biostatistics, nutrition, health planning and administration, population and family planning, and the environmental sciences. The Commission therefore believes that American schools of public health should concentrate on training selected foreign nationals in those areas at doctoral level if instruction is unavailable in their home countries. This can be facilitated by enrolling foreign students in American schools for specific specialized areas and by developing programs of systematic faculty exchange among American and foreign schools of public health and foreign medical schools, with the special objectives of training faculty and developing research competence. Such programs can be facilitated by establishing close working relationships with the World Health Organization and its regional components.

Academic centers of excellence for the specialized education of foreign nationals should be recognized, just as they should be for doctoral training of American students. These centers should be geared to meet the needs of foreign students in all appropriate subjects. Graduates of these centers would be expected to return to their own countries in teaching positions and as research scientists, to form a nucleus for the further development of professional manpower.

There is also a need to develop American career specialists in international health. Although agency demand for international health specialists is not at present great, there are positions available which go unfilled because of the lack of trained personnel. A few educational centers should train career specialists in international health problems within the multidisciplinary setting of a school of public health.

There are reciprocal benefits to the United States in concentrating scarce resources in the field of international health. Many foreign countries have paid considerable attention to evaluating their health services and to implementing innovations in delivering health services in previously unserved areas. Their methods of developing minimally trained health personnel to perform specific tasks have proved successful, and much has been learned that can be directly applied in the United States. The lessons to be learned from their experience should become part of the basic education of all public health students.

Since World War II, cooperative efforts have flourished, and the interdependence of various parts of the world in matters of public health is increasingly understood and more effectively built into continuing collaboration. Epidemiologic research—especially comparative studies of the prevalence and distribution of disease in different countries—has been of tremendous value in bringing new understanding of many diseases. Such comparisons are now being explored through the development of international collaborative research activities on such important problems as atherosclerosis, various forms of cancer, and coronary thrombosis. Moreover, the study of a disease in one country may have value for other countries even though that disease does not exist in those countries. An example is the work recently done in India on cholera, with the participation of scientists at Johns Hopkins University, which gives promise of new approaches to diarrheal disease in general. Similarly, cost-effectiveness studies of foreign experience of health services organization, emphasizing the use of specially trained ancillary personnel in developing nations, could demonstrate procedures which the more affluent countries such as the United States can emulate.

The economic value of health must be faced as a more immediately pressing question in developing countries than in industrialized nations. The relationship between the protection and improvement of health—which produces an increase in human longevity and population growth—and the economic welfare of a nation has dramatically underscored this issue. Recent population trends in many parts of the world indicate that among other things a sharp reduction in fertility may be required to balance the gains of public health measures which lower mortality rates, especially of children. As intensified and more effective health activities increase the number of children who live to maturity, economic development must be appropriately planned and coordinated with a national population policy so that the added population can be adequately nourished, educated, and housed. Public health activity must be balanced with other sectors of economic and social development. Defining methods of evaluating such change and anticipating those factors necessary to maintain or produce balanced development is crucially dependent upon the cooperation of many nations. Not only can international collaboration provide solutions to specific health problems, but it can also contribute substantially to developing those analytic and monitoring techniques necessary for effective programs of education and service.

Subjects which are particularly important in international health are environmental problems, nutrition, population dynamics, and the organization of basic health care delivery systems for the rural and urban poor. In tropical areas, which have a large part of the population of the world, recent developments suggest that the continuing massive prevalence of infectious diseases, the prospect of mass starvation, and the underlying problem of population growth are world wide challenges to implement what we already know. The availability of measures to control diseases caused by the improper disposal of human wastes, lack of safe water supply, inadequate protection of food, dangerous vectors and pollution, makes teaching and research on environmental health particularly important. The nutritional impact of the growing world food crisis, particularly for mothers and children in poor populations, is aggravated by inefficient distribution and use of available foods. All of these problems require the sort of interdisciplinary approach available through public health.

Throughout history, the effectiveness of international health measures has provided a rallying point for the development of continuing collaboration in health and for the use of health programs as models for solving other human service problems on an international scale. A striking illustration of the pivotal role of health in promoting international cooperation is found in the choice of programs by the Agency for International Development (United States State Department). In carrying out American national policy to assist developing nations, this agency has utilized the universal enthusiasm for health activities as a major component of its program planning.

As long as our government continues to be interested in providing aid to less developed countries, the Commission believes that health activities should be an important part of that effort. However, an appropriate balance should be maintained between direct assistance to foreign countries and financial support of university-based activities, so that collaborative research and education can be maintained which are of benefit to both the United States and the other countries involved.

The Commission believes that development of joint international academic consortia to bring together the complex variety of resources is essential to meaningful international health activities. We consider this approach preferable to attempts by single institutions or departments to satisfy the multiple needs of international collaborative effort, and we believe that such joint activities would help ensure the continuing quality of such undertakings.

Experience with interinstitutional arrangements involving universities in two or more countries should be evaluated in order to provide a firm basis for future planning. It should be recognized that such joint activities are especially vulnerable to funding cuts and other interruptions as a result of policy changes in one or more of the cooperating countries.

An international frame of reference in public health is especially valuable for American public health professionals to augment their own professional perspectives and to counteract provincialism through comparative analysis. In fact, it is desirable that all students in the health professions be exposed to the international dimension. A basic understanding can be obtained from an introductory course which would include, as a minimum, the international contribution to epidemiology and comparative studies of health care systems.

Recommendations

16. *Recognized centers at American schools of public health should continue to train foreign nationals in those areas of specialization for which appropriate education is not available in their home or other nearby countries. These centers should also carry out a systematic program of faculty exchange and collaborative research with foreign institutions.*

17. *Programs for the training of foreign nationals should give adequate consideration to the particular cultural, organizational, and socioeconomic needs of the individual student and/or nation.*

9. Individual Programs in Public Health Fields

We have recommended that the many programs now existing in various schools of the university be used to educate a substantial proportion of professional personnel needed for public health activities. The emphasis in these programs is necessarily task-oriented and job-related.

The key principle in relation to these programs is to make sure that the central core of the knowledge base for public health is sufficiently represented. The health professional schools must provide sufficient instruction about administration and related skills, and in the nonhealth schools there must be adequate health content. Knowledge of health problems and scientific methods is essential for everyone who is to function in the health field.

The programs of health administration in graduate schools of business or public administration now produce more than 25 percent of the graduates of special programs. These graduates are basically prepared for jobs in clinically-centered health care service organizations, rather than for the broader task of managing community health services systems, which properly devolves upon the executives or policy makers in public health. Schools of engineering give a large number of master's degrees in environmental engineering. A substantial proportion of their graduates will function directly in the health field. Schools of education and allied health give master's degrees in health education and in other fields pertinent to public health practice. Various educational institutions give graduate degrees in nutrition, and most of their graduates function as public health nutritionists.

On their own, these schools cannot be expected to be able to give sufficient public health content in the full range of the knowledge base. If students in these schools are to develop adequate comprehension of the health implications of their particular specialty, health resources not generic to the school must be involved. Currently in most such graduate programs these resources are obtained on an ad hoc basis, without an overall framework for representation of relevant elements in the program's structure. For example, many of the programs in health administration emphasize the development of administrators with too little provision of health content and orientation. Where education takes place within a specific discipline or department, the orientation of that discipline is predominant. The historical background of social policy and general principles of public health are often inadequately dealt with. Without a sufficient background in public health, the graduates of such a program may feel alienated when they try to function in a health setting after graduation.

Lack of Organizational Base

There is no doubt that a fundamental understanding of principles of organization and management, systems analysis, and economics is essential for health administration. However, the appropriate use of these principles and procedures in public health activities depends upon a thorough understanding of the issues and goals of public health, both in terms of health achievement, and of the social and political realities of the entire health services system. These programs have often been developed without clear-cut policy decisions on their place in the university. Different universities have chosen to locate them in different schools. Within similar kinds of schools they may be in different departments, and they are offered on both the graduate and undergraduate levels. The absence of an accepted organizational base for the programs has resulted in some unstable funding, because they are not firmly integrated into the total academic structure.

The quality and effectiveness of public health training depends upon the adequate and appropriate representation of all the elements in the knowledge base; both the central sciences and the cognate disciplines are needed. This requires coordination even in a curriculum aimed at the preparation of one type of professional. The problem is compounded when education is developed for one or more types of personnel in the same university, but in different professional schools or graduate departments. The challenge of organizing this effort successfully is crucial to effective education.

Where a university has or develops resources and activities to educate for public health, these must be recognized and identified as such, so that they can be mobilized to incorporate the knowledge base appropriately. There should be a responsible locus to make sure that students in a program of health administration in a business school, for example, have adequate instruction about public health. The university administration must be sure that appropriate standards and requirements are established and enforced before a degree in a public health field is awarded by any school or department.

Role of the
Academic Health Center

Many universities recognize the need for some systemization of efforts by related schools on the same campus. The academic health center or health complex has recently emerged as the predominant structure which tries to integrate disciplines and schools within individual universities, and coordinates academic health activities with social needs. Through this mechanism, all the various schools of the health professions and their related clinical facilities maintain communication and develop policy about plans and projects. This enables them to develop teaching programs which will respond to the needs of society and at the same time maximize the use of resources within the university. Although the academic health center does not of itself prevent duplication and competition in and among the different health schools, it does provide a framework for cooperative resolution of problems and the opportunity to organize activities efficiently and effectively. The Association for Academic Health Centers, established in 1971, currently lists 91 full and associate members (personal communication with AAHC, 1975).

This number indicates the rapidly growing trend toward such co-operative administrative aand organizational arrangements in our universities.

The academic health center should naturally be responsible for public health education, even when this means coordinating efforts among schools that are not part of the academic health complex. It should integrate the efforts of all contributing disciplines and departments, and help guarantee that the knowledge base is set before the students without duplication of resources or gaps in knowledge.

Need for an Administrative Focus

Where there is no academic health center organization in the university, other arrangements must be made to coordinate higher education for public health. A focus of administration for educational efforts in public health should not be an incidental, extraneous organization. It must be given the authority and responsibility to establish and maintain appropriate links between different schools and different curricula, so that all programs of higher education for public health in the university are integrated and directed to the proper academic resources for the knowledge base for public health.

Because of the interdisciplinary nature of education for public health, the responsibility for its general form cannot be left to any one school. The focus for such responsibility must be situated high enough in the university administrative structure so that access to all necessary elements can be expedited. The need for such a focus is heightened in universities which have a school of public health, as even these schools are incapable on their own of providing instruction from all disciplines, and must draw upon university resources. The lack is accentuated in single programs which emphasize a particular specialty. Frequently their directors are not adequately aware of all the essential, interdisciplinary elements of the knowledge base. A top university administrative office should be responsible for seeing that all necessary elements are represented, and for facilitating arrangements to obtain these. Where there is an office of the vice president or vice chancellor for health, this is the natural focus for that responsibility.

In addition to ensuring the provision of relevant elements of the knowledge base, this office should be responsible for seeing that appropriate arrangements are made with field agencies so that students and faculty will have close relationships with the field of practice. Currently, for example, only a small proportion (21 percent) of the programs in health and hospital administration, which confer a substantial number of master's degrees each year, have any community links, other than the residency year to enable students and faculty to make connections between academic information and its possible applications (Commission on Education for Health Administration, 1975b).

Recommendations

18. *Universities that have, or are establishing, programs designed to prepare people for public health activity, should establish an administrative focus at the highest level, next to the President, for planning and development, so as to ensure that all relevant elements of the knowledge base are appropriately represented through optimum use of university resources.*

19. *All programs of higher education for public health should have close relationships with the field of practice similar to those recommended for schools of public health, and faculty in these programs should have similar field and advocacy responsibilities.*

10. Special Responsibilities and Problems in Higher Education for Public Health

So far we have discussed our recommendations for improving the overall effort in higher education for public health in terms of the two major locations for today's efforts: the schools of public health and the various programs in other graduate schools. Each has certain general characteristics. However, there are some specific problems and responsibilities which can best be considered as applying to all public health education, no matter where it takes place. These include policies regarding minority and female students, nontraditional programs, continuing education, advocacy roles for faculty, research, and financing.

Minorities and Women

Members of minority groups—blacks, Hispanics, orientals, and native Americans—have been substantially underrepresented in public health, as they have in the other health professions. No reliable data on minority group students as a whole are available for the schools of public health except for the last two or three years. In the decade 1962 to 1972 only 3 percent of the graduates of schools of public health were black (White et al., 1974). The picture is not substantially different in other graduate school programs. For example, in 48 programs in health administration, in 1972–73, 13 percent of the enrollment were minority students. Of the total number of students, 23 percent were women (personal communication with the Association of Academic Health Centers, 1975).

In the past few years the schools of public health have made concerted efforts to correct this deficiency (Hall et al., 1973b). At the University of North Carolina, for example, minority enrollments increased from 4 percent in the academic year 1971–72 to more than 12 percent in 1973–74. In 1971 the School of Public Health at the University of California at Berkeley increased its minority enrollment from 15 to 24 percent, with a special program for American Indians (Hall et al., 1973c). The newer schools at the Universities of Texas and Illinois are also encouraging minority students. Texas reports show that in 1973 almost 20 percent of those accepted for the master's program were minority students, and at Illinois, in each of the first three entering classes, minority students constituted more than 20 percent of the student enrollment.

Although recent progress has not been sufficient to bring minority student enrollments in line with their representation in the nation as a whole, the schools of public health cannot be singled out for blame. Deficiencies in former preparation and inequalities of education at all levels decrease the numbers of qualified applicants for public health education.

Women have also been underrepresented, providing only about one-third of the student body during this period. Most female students at schools of public health have come from "sex-linked" professions such as nursing or social work. In the other part of the student body, women represent an even smaller proportion (15 percent) (Hall et al., 1973d). Affirmative action policies must obviously be pursued vigorously.

The effort to recruit students from minority groups should be expanded, not only as part of our national commitment to ensure equal opportunity and to redress historic inequities, but also to increase the effectiveness of public health efforts in the nation. Many of the health problems in the United States are most acute in minority populations. Others occur in target populations, such as mothers and children. There is reason to believe that professionals can be most effective in working with a community if they have sociocultural and/or racial backgrounds similar to those of the population they are serving. Representatives of minority groups and more women are therefore particularly needed in public health, and can make a valuable contribution to the efforts to improve and protect the health of a significant portion of our population.

Special financial support for student training will be necessary if the schools of public health are to attract enrollment from minority groups. Black and native or Spanish-speaking American families are four times more likely to have incomes below the poverty level than other American families (Office of Management and Budget, Statistical Policy Division, 1973). Because these minority students can meet a distinct national need, it seems reasonable that federal funds be made available for their support.

Recommendation

20. Federal, state, and institutional aid must be made available for minority groups and other students with substantial financial needs in order to ensure equity of access to education for public health.

Nontraditional Programs

There has been a national movement in recent years to develop special educational programs which enable people to acquire professional education in certain fields by fulfilling degree requirements without materially interrupting their employment. This is being done chiefly through night courses and off-campus teaching and/or assignments (Commission on Nontraditional Study, 1973).

Several off-campus programs in public health have been developed to offer professional degrees at the master's level to employed professionals with minimal or no on-campus time commitment. Schools of public health at the Universities of Michigan and North Carolina, at California in Berkeley and Los Angeles, Loma Linda, Hawaii, and Washington currently offer, or plan to sponsor, such degree granting programs. At present these programs are available only in health services administration; however, plans to extend this option to other fields are being contemplated. Those schools of public health now offering such off-campus, nontraditional programs are able to use regular faculty who may travel to meet students at locations in the community. The admission criteria and standards for student enrollees and course offerings are identical with those of the on-campus program. The University of North Carolina School of Public Health at Chapel Hill, for example, now offers degree programs in health administration at Raleigh, North Carolina, and at Asheville, North Carolina. A different kind of two-year work-study program is being given at the University of Michigan School of Public Health. Once a month, health administrators from the East and Middle West meet in Ann Arbor for four days of intensive classroom study. Reading assignments and special research projects are carried out during the balance of the month while the student pursues his regular job. This on-job on-campus program emphasizes administration of outpatient services, and after completion, students will receive master's degrees in public health.

During the 1975–76 academic year, the University of Cincinnati started a "University Without Walls External M.S. Degree Program in Health Planning Administration." Clusters of eight to 10 people within a given geographic area will meet three times a year for five-day sessions on campus. In between sessions the students will be provided with study guides, readings, cassettes, and other learning aids.

The off-campus programs are now financed largely by employing organizations, sponsoring universities, and demonstration grants from federal and state governments. There may be financial problems with these programs, due to federal or state funding formulas (Committee on Financing of Higher Education for Adult Students, 1974).

The value of these off-campus programs lies in their accessibility and availability to public health professionals, who are able to advance their skills and knowledge without materially interrupting their practice responsibilities. While such programs may have an important place in the education of certain public health personnel, the special problems and opportunities of such a framework need careful exploration, and could benefit from imaginative curriculum design and objective evaluation.

Continuing Education

Every health professional must be given the opportunity to update and upgrade professional knowledge and skills on a continuing basis. Increased professional and public concern for the continuing competence of health practitioners emphasizes the importance of continuing education. In addition to the manifest problem of updating professional knowledge in areas whose information base is constantly expanding, there are ever-new professional roles and functions. In every discipline the professional is confronted with new questions on ethics and personal privacy, escalating specialization, and the need for interdisciplinary approaches to problem solving. The issue of competency is particularly important to public health which has not utilized licensure or registration as a criterion for initial eligibility to practice. Generally speaking, there are no formal requirements to determine the competence of public health professionals. Often a job requirement specifies a degree or a course of study in an accredited public health or related educational program. Even this requirement is shifting as more "public health programs" are offered by academic institutions other than accredited schools of public health.

The concept of lifelong learning, especially for health professionals, brings continuing education into sharp focus and emphasizes its relationship with the rest of higher education. The term "continuing education" implies that there is an educational base from which further education takes place. This base is the formal education system which offers a range of academic programs and degrees. Continuing education may be considered to begin at whatever point a person leaves fulltime study, and the need for it continues throughout the person's life.

There are many courses and programs of continuing education in public health, sponsored by a variety of academic institutions, field agencies or professional groups. With few exceptions, however, they consist of a series of miscellaneous efforts, haphazardly conceived. They do not constitute an organized program aimed at target groups of public health professionals to fill gaps in knowledge generated by technologic developments, or identified in relation to field needs.

Several factors account for the random nature of these offerings. First, academic institutions have not accepted responsibility for providing continuing education as a comprehensive, planned program. Not enough thought has been given to who needs such education, for what specific purposes, and how each offering relates to, or complements, other offerings. Another problem has been the absence of any uniform mechanism for evaluating the quality of continuing education programs or for monitoring attendance in a relevant manner. Figures on total attendance do not give any assurance that all who need updating are in fact receiving it; and indeed, the same few may be attending many different programs, while the many remain uninstructed. Although participation by public health professionals has not been examined on a comprehensive basis, it appears that participants have demonstrated some interest in virtually every public health specialty (Hall et al., 1973e).

Little information is available regarding reasons for nonattendance. It is likely that there are fundamental problems involving lack of time, money, geographic availability, adequate advance publicity, or perhaps even lack of interest in the courses offered. For technical and managerial personnel, a variety of financial and job promotion incentives exist which are directly or indirectly related to participation in continuing education activities. For upper-level administrative personnel, however, such incentives are often either negligible or nonexistent; if these individuals are to utilize continuing education offerings, programs must meet their specific professional needs.

There are several issues which are fundamental to the effective development of continuing education for public health, notably the establishment of quality criteria for programs, and the development of mechanisms for monitoring participation and granting recognition for the completion of course units.

Recently there has been a trend in the health professions to make continuing education a component of relicensure and recertification, and a prerequisite for continued membership in professional societies. Institutional licensure, or certification, especially for public health agencies, would serve a useful function in this respect if the agencies were held responsible for monitoring and ensuring the continued professional competence of their staff. Continuing education requirements could be developed for this purpose as part of comprehensive institutional standards and review mechanisms.

The populations served by field agencies have the most to gain from adequate programs of continuing education, as the effectiveness and efficiency of personnel can be expected to increase as a result of training. The agencies should take responsibility for helping to support such programs financially, for helping to plan and design their content, and for stimulating educational institutions to provide adequate programs.

There are no standardized quality controls for continuing education in public health, and the responsibility for monitoring and revising programs has traditionally been the prerogative of the individual educational institutions. The lack of such standards has resulted in sporadic and uneven development of continuing education programs within institutions and has made comparative evaluation virtually impossible. One proposed method of standardizing current practices is the Continuing Education Unit (CEU) (National Task Force on the Continuing Education Unit, 1974). This system of accreditation and quality review, or some similar quantification, could become a nationally recognized unit for measuring individual and institutional participation in noncredit courses, programs and activities. For the individual it would serve as a yardstick of educational activity, by which eligibility for salary increments and other career benefits could be established. For the institution it would represent a unit of accounting for measuring the productivity and efficiency of their continuing education programs. The Southern and Western Associations of Colleges and Schools have already recommended the adoption of the CEU to its members. Also, some professional associations have adopted it.

Academic institutions preparing people for public health must accept continuing education as an important element in their total system of education. This cannot be done without a commitment by the university or its school of public health to an administrative focus which can serve to develop all individual efforts as relevant components of an overall program.

Recommendation

21. *In all institutions providing higher education for public health, continuing education should occupy a distinct and prominent role in the program:*
    (1) *There should be a clearly defined focus of responsibility for academic and administrative components.*
    (2) *Coherent programs should be developed to fill identified gaps in knowledge for target groups of professionals.*
    (3) *Basic standardized national criteria should be developed to ensure quality of course offerings, and to facilitate the systematic recording of individual and institutional participation in programs of continuing education.*

Advocacy

Professional involvement in public health carries with it the commitment to see that scientific knowledge is put to broad, effective use. Educators in programs of higher education for public health have a responsibility to see that relevant information is shared with the public, so that public cooperation can be obtained to stimulate the actions needed to solve major health problems. When faculty members have responsibilities for field activity, they should use their expertise to develop public understanding of major health issues. This may, on occasion, entangle them in political or otherwise controversial issues, as public health programs compete with other social needs for public resources. No faculty member should have to draw back from engagement because he fears to compromise his institution or some mythical neutrality of academe.

The history of public health in the United States is full of examples of professionals who fought diligently and courageously to convince the public to take needed, and perhaps unpleasant or costly, action to control communicable diseases. The shift in the nature of public health problems to environmental concerns and effective delivery of personal health services has found official public health agencies unready and to some extent unwilling to undertake these responsibilities effectively. Organized academic programs in public health have been important sources of research and training in these areas. However, the faculties, as such, in concentrating on their academic work, have not fostered their relationship with the field of practice and with the general public.

There is a great need for professional courage to confront the major health problems of today, and we suggest that there are good reasons for public health faculties providing the necessary leadership. They can be expected to have the appropriate expertise, and the fact that they are not directly accountable to voters or political pressures not only protects them but also gives their advice a useful quality of impartiality and objectivity. Active advocacy, like other forms of service, together with teaching and research, should be weighed for faculty promotion.

Recommendation

22. Educational institutions preparing people for public health should expect faculty members to serve as informed advocates of effective health policies, programs, and practices, and firmly support them even if such advocacy becomes controversial.

Research

Research is fundamental to effective public health activity and education. While some research is done in most programs of higher education for public health, by far the largest portion of that activity is carried on by the schools of public health. The Commission therefore queried these schools about the nature and scope of their research programs, and the auspices and sources of financial support. Thirteen schools responded of the 18 queried, and this sample was representative of all the schools in terms of the size of the research effort.

During the academic year 1973–74 more than 400 separate studies were being conducted in the 13 reporting schools. These studies covered a wide range of subjects, which can be catergorized as shown in the following list. (These categories are not mutually exclusive and certain studies may fit into two or more of the categories.)

   —Research on specific diseases—epidemiologic and biomedical studies
   —Research on the organization of personal health services—
   —studies of manpower, financing, planning, and utilization patterns
   —Research on environmental factors—noise, air and water pollutants, and solid wastes; health effects; and control technology
   —Research methodology—development, evaluation, and refinement of techniques and tools.

There is little duplication of studies either within or among the 13 schools reporting. This is noteworthy, considering the fragmentation of sources of funding for the research. More than 40 federal funding agencies and more than 20 different foundations and voluntary organizations support research projects in these schools of public health. Several dozen other projects are supported by state and local governments and by labor unions or industries.

The total currently allocated from all sources for this research is about $75,000,000. This amount is budgeted over periods ranging from one to five years. Eighty-five percent of these funds comes directly or indirectly from institutes, departments, or bureaus of the federal government. Six percent comes from foundations and voluntary organizations, with the balance from various other sources. The federal government grants average more than $200,000 per study, with a range from $7,500 to over four million dollars per study. Nonfederal sources give considerably less for each research project.

There is a considerable range in the amount of research funding allocated to the different schools. The Harvard School of Public Health lists grants amounting to $20,000,000, which accounts for more than 25 percent of the research funds for all 13 schools. The newer schools report research grants totalling $2,000,000 or less per school.

Faculty interest, competency, and reputation play an important role in attracting financial support for research. For example, five of the eight current research projects at the University of Illinois School of Public Health (a new school) are concerned with environmental health. The presence of one faculty member at this school may well be an important reason for this emphasis on environmental health studies, as this faculty member is the principal investigator for two projects which account for more than 75 percent of all funds currently granted for research in that institution.

Similarly, at the University of California at Los Angeles School of Public Health, eight of the research projects are nutritional studies and one faculty member is the principal investigator in six of these. There are three major projects of specific research, on obstructive respiratory disease, multiple sclerosis, and hypertension, which account for over $1,000,000 or 20 percent of the total funds for research at this school. One faculty member is the principal investigator in all three projects. Another faculty member specializes in survey research and is principal investigator in three projects at UCLA which account for nearly 25 percent of the school's total research grants.

Harvard is still another example where in spite of considerable diversity, five faculty members account for well over $11,000,000 or about half of the total research funds at that school. One faculty member is principal investigator in four projects in tropical public health, another is responsible for three projects in epidemiology, two faculty members share four projects in physiology, and another is principal investigator in three general research projects which alone account for more than 20 percent of Harvard's total research funds in public health.

While most of the research in these schools is diversified (by subject matter, methodology, and objectives), several schools concentrate efforts in one sector or another. Faculty competence in a given research area of course attracts support for specific types of research. In addition, the geographic location of a given school of public health sometimes affects the research emphasis.

The great increase in the 1960s in federal support for research in public health, as in other health fields, has had a significant effect on the nature of the research done in the schools. Often it has meant that subjects for research are chosen because funds have been available for the study of a particular subject. While the federal research funds have often supported faculty members who can then contribute to the teaching efforts of the institution, this has also meant that the federal government has been setting research priorities in the academic institution. This is not always bad, as it sometimes results in research that is realistically related to the needs and interests of the nation. However, priorities may be determined by political pressures, not always reflecting the priorities as perceived by scientists in the field. Such was considered to be the case with the recent establishment of the national "all-out attack on cancer," which many medical and public health experts considered a distortion of priorities in biomedical research. This view was taken not because cancer is unimportant, but because predicating support for research on its relevance to cancer contravenes the established principle that it is often difficult to predict the ultimate value of fundamental research in relation to specific diseases.

Research done in schools of public health contributes to the objectives of these schools, if only because all research on public health subjects can be expected to make some contribution to the depth of the academic effort. However, the schools have had little opportunity to determine an overall research policy themselves. In general it has been assumed that research plans and proposals must, perforce, be developed by faculty members themselves, either individually or in small groups, as good research depends upon their skills, knowledge, and creativity. Thus, the research activities of a school represent the sum of a series of individual projects, influenced by the expressed interest of funding agencies, particularly by the U.S. Department of Health, Education, and Welfare.

Without denying the reality of how good research is developed and conducted, it would be desirable for research efforts in a school to reflect the predominant mission of that school and of its faculty. The provision of research funds for specific projects, either as grants or contracts, sometimes makes this difficult. In recent years the proportion of funds supplied through contracts has increased. This restricts the ability of schools and faculty to develop research activities which directly reflect the basic interest and mission of the schools. General research funds support, for the development of pilot projects, has been reduced sharply in recent years.

The practice of some funding agencies to support research programs and centers in broad areas, such as cancer, cardiovascular disease, or health services, presents an opportunity for developing research in relation to an institution's basic mission and interest. Selection of institutions for this type of support is made on the basis of resources and demonstrated competence of faculty, and gives freedom and flexibility in the choice of specific projects within the overall framework of a research program. Support for research programs and centers, as distinguished from individual projects and contracts has additional advantages. Financial support is provided for a longer period of time, generally five years, with decisions about continued funding for another cycle made well in advance of the termination of current funding. Thus an institution can plan more realistically for faculty and related resources.

Schools of public health should develop plans which would outline the components of a research program consistent with the predominant mission of the school. This would increase each school's ability to use a wide range of funding possibilities. A plan has obvious advantages over the present system where each opportunity is grasped as it appears, on the theory that some research is always better than none.

With full knowledge of the practical difficulties involved in implementing any plan to coordinate research, the Commission still believes that special attention should be given to the development of research which is relevant to the region in which a school is located. For example, Columbia University's school of public health, located in New York City, tends to emphasize urban health problems, such as alcoholism, drug abuse, and the high prevalence of emotional illness. This concentration is organically related to that school's opportunities and commitment. If community-oriented research efforts are made in collaboration with local operating agencies, providers, and consumers, an excellent opportunity is provided for the strengthening of faculty and student relationships with the field. This would further serve to help integrate research into the learning process.

In addition to its substantive value, research is, of course, a necessary part of the educational experience for both faculty and students. It is useful for faculty members in that it can aid in the development of new teaching material as well as help them to continue their professional growth. Students at the master's level can gain an appreciation of the methods, skills, and the rewards of research by observation of, and participation in, projects underway at the school. For students at the doctoral level, faculty research offers a context in which to do their own independent studies by extending or relating to the departmental research topics.

Health-related issues often extend beyond specific professional fields, and it may sometimes be difficult to define those which are clearly proper subjects for research in a school of public health. But criteria should be developed before a school commits a substantial portion of its faculty energies and physical resources to a project. Such research would be expected to contribute to a better understanding of problems in public health. These problems should also be ones that cannot be dealt with elsewhere with equal effectiveness. In the search for biologic measures to prevent poliomyelitis, for example, all of the laboratory work could have been—and in fact much of it was—carried out in medical schools. The unique contributions of the public health approach were seen in the field trials which were used to evaluate the effectiveness of the vaccines developed in the laboratory. These two aspects of the research efforts on one subject demonstrate the unique character of public health research as contrasted to general medical or biologic research. This is not to say that no basic biologic research should be done in the school of public health. But the research skills and knowledge involved in the field trial activity are uniquely generic to public health and should therefore be emphasized by public health faculties. Other issues which specifically require public health approaches would include studies on the evaluation of the quality of medical care, certain aspects of occupational or environmental health, the epidemiology of chronic disease, and the design of large-scale or long-term studies to identify causative factors in disease or evaluate the efficacy of therapeutic measures.

While it might be argued that there is more knowledge and technology already available to health professionals throughout the world than they are at present able to deliver through intervention programs, it is also true that there are important gaps. Indeed, the very failure to translate knowledge into action is itself a matter that demands intensive research.

Current programs in health education of the community and in the training of professionals to plan, organize, carry out, and evaluate these efforts suffer from the lack of basic knowledge necessary to achieve the desired goal of producing changes in health-related behavior. For many years the attempt to produce behavioral change with regard to health, focused on the dissemination of more and more attractively presented information. The American public has been saturated with health information—in the newspapers, magazines, on television, and through special leaflets and pamphlets put out by health agencies. However, factual information alone has not succeeded in bringing about desired behavioral changes to any significant extent. The recognition of this failure has important implications for all of public health.

What people will do about their health depends on social and cultural, as well as disease-specific, factors. In addition, their behavior is based not so much on the amount or type of knowledge that they have as on attitudes towards life-style, health, and health services. It has long been accepted that sociodemographic variables such as age, sex, social class, and ethnic group identification play major roles in determining receptivity to health education messages, utilization of health services, participation in screening programs, and reaction to symptoms and treatment. In addition, psychologic, sociologic, and economic factors are important, and these must be understood before information can be given to people so that it will be used in a meaningful manner. However, the incorporation of the contributions of the various social sciences into the training of health educators does not seem to have solved the problem of motivating people to make behavioral changes.

Breast cancer is a graphic example of the inadequacy of current efforts in health education of the public. The effectiveness and importance of screening methods and self-examination for early detection of breast cancer have been known for several decades, yet it was recently shown that only a small proportion of the women at risk participate in such activities. Then, in the autumn of 1974, the wife of the president of the United States underwent surgery for breast cancer and there was widespread publicity about her mastectomy. Within a few days facilities for mammography were swamped with requests for examination. Obviously, something happened in the minds and hearts of women reading about the First Lady which moved them to act, although they had ignored previous professional attempts to get them to do this. It is true that a crisis or a dramatic tragedy is often necessary to stimulate change, but surely it should be possible for professionals to develop equally productive alternatives?

The potential for community self-education must also be explored. Patient organizations or self-help groups, usually identified with a common disease or social problem (e.g., Alcoholics Anonymous, Weight Watchers, individuals with colostomies or mastectomies) have established the unique and valuable contribution that can be made by cooperative self-help efforts. Through sharing techniques of self-care, as well as providing empathy and support for others in similar circumstances, individuals in these groups gain health knowledge, help to publicize the concepts of preventive health behavior, and sometimes are able to achieve behavioral change where exhortation or persuasion from health professionals has failed.

The schools of public health have much to contribute in this difficult area of health education. They possess both the interdisciplinary resources and the interest in the subject necessary to undertake research in this field. The Commission believes that the schools of public health have a unique responsibility here and should undertake as a major endeavor, to develop research which will lead to effective programs of health education.

Research in public health needs organization and unifying foci. In speaking of these issues, the Commission does not mean to suggest that research tasks be dictated or that academic freedom be curbed. In fact, for some time, many individual and institutional research choices have been dominated by funding practices. It is now time for discussion which may lead to a conceptual framework in which decisions about emphasis in research can be made in ways which would relate programs of research more directly to the ultimate goals of public health.

An institutional plan for research should deal not only with the substance of research, but also with the scale of research, the general characteristics of research, and the terms and conditions under which federal funds are provided. Scale is important because research should not be permitted to grow so large that teaching is impaired. The characteristics of research, such as the intellectual challenge of the work, are important because they affect the inevitability of the research in an academic setting. Terms and conditions are important because sponsors sometimes undertake to impose conditions which threaten the autonomy of the institution.

Without attempting to provide a definitive list of subjects, the Commission offers a few examples of newer problems which deserve consideration on any agenda of public health research:

—How can values of health and well-being be introduced into policy decisions of potential health importance which lie outside the jurisdiction of public health authorities?

—How can people be motivated to change their life-styles and to accept and apply proven means for protecting their physical and mental health?

—What is the best method for the early discovery and surveillance of environmental health hazards?

—What are the possible tradeoffs between economic stability or growth and protection against health hazards?

—How can a more equitable distribution of personnel, facilities, and programs be developed?

Research is a vital element in the teaching and service of all programs of higher education in public health. Indeed higher education cannot thrive or be effective without it. Although much of this discussion has centered on the research efforts of the schools of public health, we feel it is also essential for graduate programs of education for public health in other schools of the university to engage in research within the purview of their special focus, so that their curricula can be enriched and the boundaries of public health knowledge enlarged.

Recommendation

23. *A sustained and heightened research effort is needed in all graduate programs providing higher education for public health.*

The schools of public health have special opportunities to focus their unique interdisciplinary perspective and resources on the development of research, both applied and basic, on a wide range of present and emerging public health problems.

Financing

Any approach to the question of financing higher education for public health must first distinguish between the efforts in the schools of public health and those located elsewhere in the university. Specialty programs, such as those in health care administration and health planning now offered by schools of public administration, schools of business, etc., must be considered properly in the context of the financing of the schools in which they are located. Because these programs are established as incremental efforts in operating schools, they require only a few additional faculty responsible solely for the program. Existing courses in the school can be used, and faculty already available may develop additional courses. However, their contribution of operating level personnel should be recognized by government sources when funding for public health manpower is contemplated.

Schools of public health now supply approximately half the trained personnel for public health activities in the nation. A sound financial basis for their operations is therefore an essential part of the national public health effort. The problem of finding an adequate and firm financial base is particularly complex and serious for these schools. The cost of education in schools of public health is as expensive as the most costly professional education, with approximately the same amount spent per student per year as in medical education, although the total cost per student is less because the period of study is shorter in most instances (Institute of Medicine, National Academy of Sciences, 1974; personal communication with Ruth Hanft, 1974).

As with everything else, there has been a great change in costs in schools of public health over the past 25 years. The manner in which schools meet these costs has also undergone great changes. In

1949–50, when there were nine schools of public health with 1,239 students, total expenditure including research was approximately $4.8 million for all schools. Eighteen percent of the funds were from federal sources and were earmarked for research only (Rosenfeld et al., 1953).

The most significant change in the pattern of funding of schools of public health in the past quarter century has been their growing dependence on federal funds. Substantial federal involvement began in 1956 with the provision of traineeships for students in specialized areas, to encourage training relevant to national needs. Under the Hill-Rhodes Act of 1958 the federal government began to supply formula grants for general educational support, as distinct from categorical program support (U.S. Public Health Service Act #309 (c), 1958; U.S. Public Health Service Act #309 (a), 1958).

Beginning in 1960, project grants were awarded competitively to strengthen and expand training of public health professionals in specialized fields. Table 6 summarizes these appropriations on a yearly basis. It can be seen that, from the relatively small amount of one million dollars first provided in 1957, federal financing of the schools of public health rapidly increased over the next 10 years and remained roughly at this level. Legislative authority for this funding has now expired, and support has been provided under a continuing resolution.

State funds were also increased over this period, and several new schools were opened. Programs were expanded, faculty enlarged, and student enrollment increased markedly. By 1972 there were 18 schools of public health (seven at private and 11 at public universities) with 5,320 students enrolled and with total expenditures, including research, for all schools (1970–71) of $83,478,400 (Richardson, 1973a). There is a range of expenditures by the different schools which is not solely related to the number of students enrolled. Thus the largest school in terms of enrollment had an operating budget of almost 7 million dollars while the fifth largest had one of over 14 million dollars. Three of the 17 schools account for 40 percent of the total expenditures by schools of public health.

The range of expenditures at the schools varies widely among the different divisions and departments. For the year 1970–71, if the

Table 6

Federal Appropriations
(In Dollars)

Fiscal Year Ending	Traineeships[1]	Project Grants[2]	Formula Grants[3]
1957	1,000,000	—————	—————
1958	2,000,000	—————	—————
1959	2,000,000	—————	450,000
1960	2,000,000	—————	1,000,000
1961	2,000,000	1,430,000	1,000,000
1962	2,000,000	2,000,000	1,900,000
1963	4,000,000	2,000,000	1,900,000
1964	4,195,000	2,000,000	1,900,000
1965	4,500,000	2,500,000	2,500,000
1966	7,000,000	4,000,000	3,500,000
1967	8,000,000	5,000,000	3,750,000
1968	8,000,000	4,500,000	4,000,000
1969	8,000,000	4,917,000	4,554,000
1970	8,000,000	4,917,000	4,554,000
1971	8,400,000	4,517,000	5,054,000
1972	8,400,000	4,517,000	5,554,000
1973			
President's Budget	9,000,000	6,000,000	5,940,000
Revised Budget	9,000,000		5,940,000
1974 (President)			
1974 (House)	9,600,000	0	0

[1] Section 306—traineeship support, General Purpose (schools of public health only). Special Purpose, short-term training programs, and certain other specialized programs.

[2] Section 309(a)—project grants for institutional support for programs judged to be especially needed, open to any nonprofit institution or agency.

[3] Section 309(c)—formula grant; total sum divided among all accredited schools of public health, one-third equally and two-thirds in proportion to federally sponsored students.

Source: Personal communication from the Bureau of Health Manpower, Department of Health, Education, and Welfare.

total funds for all schools are examined as a group and distributed among the areas of expenditure, it is clear that the largest amount expended was in epidemiology, with health services administration a close second. This covers expenditures for all purposes, including research and teaching. Expenditures in epidemiology and infectious disease accounted for 22 percent of the total spent, followed by, health services administration with 21 percent; environmental health with 15 percent, population studies with 12 percent, general administration with 11 percent, nutrition with 5 percent, and biostatistics with 5 percent (Richardson, 1973b).

Table 7

1970-71 Fiscal Schema Data for Schools of Public Health[1] by Sources of Funds
(Expenditure Data: Percentage Distribution Within Each School)

School	Institutional Funds	Training and Teaching Grants and Contracts		Research Grants and Contracts		Service Grants and Contracts		Totals
		Federal	All Other	Federal	All Other	Federal	All Other	
01	9.7	38.5	9.1	1.0	6.0	35.7	—	100.00
02	26.5	18.7	1.1	39.2	13.8	—	—	100.00
03	17.2	27.4	2.6	49.5	3.2	—	—	100.00
04	20.2	31.0	0.9	37.9	6.5	—	3.5	100.00
05	20.2	34.7	2.8	38.3	2.9	—	1.1	100.00
06	14.9	18.9	—	58.3	7.4	—	—	100.00
07	26.1	37.7	0.9	30.1	5.2	—	—	100.00
08	27.0	35.8	0.6	29.5	7.1	—	—	100.00
09	16.1	39.8	2.5	37.1	1.8	—	2.7	100.00
10	15.9	21.3	0.1	40.7	3.9	—	18.1	100.00
11	49.6	36.8	0.6	9.0	2.1	—	1.9	100.00
12	51.7	9.2	—	32.7	5.6	—	0.8	100.00
13	23.9	37.9	0.1	27.8	2.1	8.1	0.1	100.00
14	63.8	12.2	—	—	—	12.6	11.4	100.00
15	17.9	52.5	1.5	26.9	1.2	—	—	100.00
16	30.1	47.2	3.5	6.2	2.1	—	10.9	100.00
17	27.5	11.9	—	60.6	—	—	—	100.00
Totals	23.0	30.0	1.2	36.8	5.5	1.7	1.8	100.00

[1] Available for 17 schools only for that period.

Source: Richardson, A.H., "Report on the Fiscal Scheme Study for the ASPH-BHME Contract," May 1973. Unpublished.

The marked dependence of the schools on federal funds in 1970–71 can be seen in Table 7. More than two-thirds of total funding derived from federal sources, although among the schools there is a range of dependence from 25 percent in one school to almost 80 percent in another. Most schools derived more than two-thirds of their total budgets from various federal funding mechanisms. Only three schools used institutional funds for half or more of their total operating budgets, while one school covered less than 10 percent of its expenses from institutional funds. The funds include state appropriations for state universities, and account for only 23 percent of total funding. Even in schools under private control only 23 percent of faculty salaries are paid by institutional funds, with nearly all the remainder supported by federal and other grants.

The proportion of separately funded research increased only from 31 percent to 42 percent of total expenditures between 1949–50 and 1970–71, although the absolute amount in dollars increased greatly (Rosenfeld et al., 1953; Richardson, 1973a). Faculty members supported by research funds commonly spend a portion of their time teaching students. Equipment purchased for research projects also can contribute to the teaching program of a school. Thus the distribution of research funds affects the quality and emphases of the teaching programs. With more than 85 percent of the research at schools of public health funded by agencies of the federal government, the effect of federal policies on the schools is profound.

This extreme dependence on federal funds has placed the schools in a precarious position. Since January 1973, the federal government has changed its policies for the financing of education for the health professions. Various federal budgets for 1974 proposed decreases of from 28 percent to 43 percent in support of nonresearch activities in the schools of public health. While some of these funding cuts have been temporarily restored, it is unlikely that in the foreseeable future federal funds will flow as readily to the schools as they have in the past. This makes it difficult for them to plan a consistent program of education for the future. Their ability to devise balanced programs of education is also affected by the large proportion of funds restricted for categorical use through the mechanism of either a research or a project grant. Today, all universities face severe economic constraints. In view of this we believe that approaches to the financial problems of the schools must concentrate on selective containment of costs, and realignment and stabilization of sources of funding, in addition to generating new sources of income where possible. In fact, many of the recommendations made so far emphasize reorganization and rearrangements which would effectively avoid waste and expensive duplication of resources, while contributing to the quality of education.

Adoption of the new mission suggested for the schools, which emphasizes the education of specified groups and more selective admission policies, would have a major impact on the economy of the schools. Some special programs would be eliminated or reduced in size, as would special courses designed to compensate for deficiences in the preparation of entering students.

We find that there are far too many courses offered in the schools today, many with only two, three, or five students in a class. There can be no justification for such faculty-student ratios in training programs at the master's level. A central reason for this proliferation of courses has been the proliferation of departments and programs, some of which should be eliminated. With fewer departments, courses duplicating others within the schools could be eliminated. The use of other departments in the university to provide instruction at the schools will also conserve funds, as this cuts down the need for special full-time faculty.

The Commission is well aware that programs are not easily started and stopped. Many tenured faculty members are supported by project grants or "soft money." Eliminating a course or a department does not eliminate the tenure obligation, nor does it erase the often real and satisfactory service a faculty member has rendered in the past. However, we reiterate that merely because a step is difficult, that does not mean it should not be taken.

The university administration should be involved in working out arrangements to minimize dislocations. Faculty members who have been engaged in training operating level personnel in a school of public health might be relocated in a graduate program for that purpose in another school of the same university. A department of social science might absorb faculty in their discipline from the school of public health if these departments begin to function as a source of instruction for the school. There are various courses of action for any university to take, given the determination to implement a new policy.

The schools will still need stable support, and federal funding is crucial if the schools are to fulfill their mission in terms of the national need in addition to exercising themselves to attain efficiency and economy. Schools of public health, like schools of medicine, prepare people who will contend with life and death issues for all Americans. The education of professional personnel for leadership in executive functions, the development of biostatisticians and epidemiologists, researchers, and educators in public health constitutes an important national resource. It is then logical for the federal government to support the schools of public health to achieve these ends.

Funding will also be needed for the programs of education for public health in other graduate schools of the university. When these programs are specifically designed to meet national manpower needs, federal project grants should be available to them. However, the major purpose of these programs is understood to be the preparation of professional personnel predominantly for state and local agencies, and voluntary organizations. State support is essential if these programs are to fulfill their mandate. Where state universities have a school of public health, the state should begin to work toward an altered mode of preparation for public health manpower. If the school concentrates on the mission we have suggested, we would anticipate a probable decrease in the school's enrollment, as some types of students at present enrolled would be diverted to other graduate programs. This would automatically cut state funding to the school of public health, as in many states support is based upon enrollment. State funds would therefore be available and could be diverted for the primary purpose of training operating level personnel. Ultimately, it might be expected that the bulk of state funds would go to support programs of higher education for public health in other graduate schools. This shift in funding sources may in the long run prove beneficial for the schools of public health. Their current financial problems do not stem from the numbers of students enrolled but in part from the fact that state governments do not recognize the high cost of public health education when allotting state funds to a school. Funding per individual student is usually inadequate. Broad, basic support would help compensate for the low budget allotment per full-time equivalent (FTE) from state funds or from basic budgets in private universities.

A period of time will be necessary during which the school of public health makes adjustments leading to implementation of its own new role and policies, and during which a realignment of federal and state support takes place. This will have to be worked out carefully, with firm commitments from both state and federal governments, to ensure that no school or program is left without needed funds during this period.

Virtually all graduates of educational programs for public health enter some form of public service. This was the major rationale in the past for federal financial support of students at schools of public health. In 1970, more than 50 percent of these students received such support. In the past few years, however, federal support of students has been sharply cut, as it was considered unnecessary if enough students of adequate quality were matriculating without federal stipends. With this decline in federal support there has been no decline in the number or quality of applications to schools of public health to date. However, the changes we recommend in the role of the schools and in their admission policies may alter the situation.

It remains to be seen how admissions to the schools of public health will be affected. Applicants who have prior degrees or years of field experience would necessarily be applying at older ages and will probably forego substantial income. If there are serious problems in attracting such students, an increase in general student support funds from the federal government will be essential. We therefore urge careful attention to this complex problem, although we do not recommend an increase in federal support for students in public health at this time. Except for special forms of assistance for students from deprived groups, the whole question of student support is a matter of general national policy. We do not feel that a special case can be made at this time for graduate students in public health as distinct from other graduate students.

The Commission believes that a variety of work-study relationships adds to the educational experience and broadens the sources of general student support. As competition for places in professional programs increases and support is more difficult to obtain, we believe students will be more and more willing to use other means of underwriting their education. Assistantship and research positions are traditional work-study methods used to support graduate students in other fields. This principle should be expanded to community agencies and institutions, which would provide students with financial support in return for work to be done either concurrently with the academic program or in alternating periods away from campus or as a job commitment from the student after graduation (with repayment provisions in case of student default).

While health agencies have traditionally arranged for capable employees to return to school for graduate training at full salary, schools and programs might explore some variations on this theme. For example, a rural program with difficulty in attracting staff might be able to hire a prospective graduate student for one year, who would promise a year's work after graduate training.

In addition, better sources of loans are needed with longer periods for repayment than are conventionally given by banks (Dresch, 1974). The Commission agrees with the recommendations regarding guaranteed student loans and national direct student loans recently made by the American Council on Education (Saunders, 1975). Universities involved in education for public health should explore with relevant professional associations, the establishment of a student revolving loan fund deferring payment until after graduation, with repayment based on a fixed percentage of income.

Stable and augmented financial support of higher education for public health is essential. In addition to systematic long-term federal support, a series of measures has been suggested which includes aggressive pursuit of new support sources through contract relationships with state governments, regional compacts, and institutional reorganization for faculty and departmental efficiency and economy. The following recommendations are made with the full awareness that they are interdependent.

Recommendations

24. *There is a distinct and continuous national need for people who will function as executives, planners, policy makers and leaders in the field of public health, epidemiologists, biostatisticians, research scientists, and educators. Therefore, the schools of public health should receive continuous basic support from the federal government to carry out educational programs to satisfy this need.*

25. *State governments should provide—as some do now—financial support for all graduate programs which prepare people for public health activity at the operating level in state and local public health programs.*

26. *Academic institutions responding to national needs for specific types of public health manpower should receive federal grant support for that purpose. This support, should, of course, be time-limited where this is appropriate in terms of the estimate of national need*

11. Related Professional Schools:

•

Medicine, Nursing, Dentistry, Veterinary Medicine, Pharmacy, Optometry, Podiatry

Ultimately, all health professionals spend a portion of their professional time in activities which are, or should be, related to public health. Their contributions can be significantly increased, and communication with public health strengthened, if their education is designed to provide a greater understanding of the concepts and methods on which these activities depend.

Greater emphasis on public health during the basic professional education of students in schools of medicine, nursing, dentistry, pharmacy, veterinary medicine, optometry, and podiatry, is essential to increase practitioners' understanding, use, and support of public health programs, enhance their own effectiveness in clinical practice, and generate interest in public health in an effort to recruit health professionals for specialization in this field.

Medical Schools

Physicians were once the predominant professionals active in public health. Over the years, as public health activities have expanded and changed, a variety of other professionals has been recruited into the field, and the relative proportion of physicians has declined. The Commission finds, however, that physicians continue to be crucial to public health activities as leaders whose comprehensive background and professional prestige accord them a unique influence. Also, their clinical knowledge and competence provide the base for advanced work in such fields as epidemiology and environmental health, in the organization of specific health care programs, and in research in the organization and evaluation of the quality of medical care.

Unfortunately, for many reasons public health is not a popular medical specialty. Medical education concentrates on the pathophysiology of disease and on the diagnosis and treatment of the sick patient, and places less emphasis on community and environmental aspects of health and disease. Medical and surgical specialties tend to dominate the power structure of medical schools, with community health or preventive medicine having comparatively little influence. Although this situation has begun to change in recent years, the effect in most schools has not been marked.

Public health and preventive medicine are represented as a distinct section of the examination given by the National Board of Medical Examiners. In spite of this official recognition, the subjects are not allotted major amounts of time in the curriculum, and there is little doubt that the section is considered of relatively minor importance by the students.

Medical students have little contact with public health practice, with public health physicians, or with attractive role models in preventive medicine and public health. Their experience in medical school is not the only factor discouraging students from entering the field of public health: the private practice of medicine today offers far greater monetary rewards and community status than does a public health position. Medical schools cannot escape responsibility for preparing physicians for their community role and must contribute to the education of physicians for this purpose. To accomplish this, medical school faculties must strengthen teaching in the fundamentals of public health, epidemiology, biostatistics, and the community-wide environmental and social aspects of health. Emphasis on health promotion and disease prevention can also be expected to increase the effectiveness of all future physicians, no matter what area of specialization they elect. Although most medical schools require at least some course work in epidemiology, biostatistics, and medical care during the first two years of study (Association of Teachers of Preventive Medicine, 1974) and many offer electives in public health areas, these teaching programs need

Table 8

Type of Courses Currently Offered to Medical Students
Expressed as Percent of Departments Responding Affirmatively[1]
(Required and Elective)

	Freshman		Sophomore		Junior		Senior		At least 1 Required
Course	R	E	R	E	R	E	R	E	course
Epidemiology	26	10	52	23	2	17	2	33	74
Biostatistics	35	12	28	19	3	15	0	27	58
Medical care	34	20	39	30	6	19	6	39	65
Other disciplines	25	18	20	25	8	18	1	31	45
Clerkships	8	8	2	14	16	28	12	61	31

[1] Data from 88 medical schools (80 percent) which responded to a survey conducted by the Association of Teachers of Preventive Medicine, Fall 1973.

Source: Association of Teachers of Preventive Medicine, 1974 Newsletter 21, No. 1.

to be expanded (Table 8). Though recently, interest in strengthening teaching in these fields has been expressed by some medical faculties, there are only a few medical schools where this has occurred to any significant extent.

Recommendation

27. Because a medical education will continue to provide many professionals with a basic foundation for important responsibilities in public health, medical schools should provide more emphasis on such subjects as epidemiology, preventive medicine, the organization, delivery and evaluation of health care, and environmental health concerns.

During the past 10 years a great deal of attention has been given to primary care and family medicine. In the minds of many people the two terms are interchangeable, but in fact they represent somewhat different things. Primary care includes preventive, diagnostic, maintenance, and remedial care. It is conceived of as providing entry into the medical care system for the patient as well as continuity and comprehensiveness of personal medical care services. Today, this type of care is provided primarily by an internist, pediatrician or a family physician. Family medicine is a new term which emphasizes primary care and deals with the family as a whole, rather than just the individual. During the past 10 years departments of family practice have been established in 75 medical schools (American Academy of Family Physicians, 1974), and there has been a corollary development of residency programs in family practice at 164 hospitals (Division of Medical Education, 1973).

The federal government has been particularly active in promoting development of this field. National interest in such programs is based at least partially upon the hope that this development will to some extent produce a redistribution of physicians, so that more of them will be available in sparsely settled, and inner-city areas. However, there is little evidence that this type of redistribution or redeployment can be expected simply because physicians are trained to practice primary care or family medicine.

Medical schools have used several models in developing their family medicine programs. Some have set up autonomous clinical departments at the same level as other clinical departments. Others have left the development of programs to departments of medicine or pediatrics, or have arranged for several clinical departments such as medicine, pediatrics, obstetrics, and psychiatry cooperatively to develop programs which function as a unit dependent upon the parent departments. Fifteen medical schools have integrated family medicine with the department of community medicine or department of preventive medicine and public health (American Academy of Family Physicians, 1974).

This last arrangement appears to reflect an assumption that family medicine or primary care carry special community health responsibilities. It also reflects another assumption, that they really represent community and preventive medicine per se. This latter concept is erroneous. Not only are the skills and knowledge of the community health specialist different from those necessary for the practice of family medicine, but also the basic philosophic approach, perspective, attitudes, and tasks undertaken are different.

While preventive medicine is relevant to every clinical specialty, it is in itself a specialized field of medicine whose primary focus is health and disease as these occur in communities and defined population groups. Its aim is to promote practices which will advance health, prevent disease, make possible early diagnosis and treatment, and foster rehabilitation of those with disabilities. In addition to general clinical sciences, its basic disciplines include biostatistics, epidemiology, administration, and the social and biomedical sciences.

This integration of family and community medicine tends to obscure the identity of community medicine and may result in dilution of preventive medicine teaching for medical students. It is important to preserve a separate identity for community medicine as taught in medical schools, if the little instruction in public health that medical students now receive is not to be weakened further.

Recommendation

28. *The current status of the teaching of community health in medical schools should be reviewed, and strong positive programs to correct deficiencies should be developed. The Association of American Medical Colleges should take the leadership for this review together with other organizations such as the Association of Schools of Public Health, the Association of Teachers of Preventive Medicine, the Association of Academic Health Centers, the American Board of Preventive Medicine, and the American College of Preventive Medicine.*

There are 62 postgraduate medical residency programs in preventive medicine—26 in general preventive medicine, 24 in public health, eight in occupational medicine and four in aerospace medicine. These programs require two years of supervised practice and at least one year of academic study. There are 13 medical schools involved in these residency programs. However, the academic portion is carried out predominantly at schools of public health (Division of Medical Education, 1973).

Most residency programs in medicine and surgery are supported largely by the patient care budget of the participating hospital. These budgets and those of other service programs are simply not available for funding residencies in preventive medicine. Federal financial support for residencies in preventive medicine and public health has been supplied since 1966 in the form of traineeships. These were awarded to schools of public health and other public or nonprofit institutions providing graduate or specialized training in public or community health. Individual award recipients have been determined by the institution. Eight schools of public health and 11 medical schools have participated in this support since 1968 (Bureau of Health Resources Development, 1974a).

In recent years there has been a marked reduction in funds authorized for these traineeships (Bureau of Health Resources Development, 1974b). In 1973 all funds were impounded and while some were later released, the current level of funding for traineeships is still well below the 1972 peak period.

Residency programs for public health must at least be financially competitive with other residency programs if they are to attract medical graduates. Strong links between medical school and residency programs will also make it easier for students to enter such programs. A commitment by a medical school to strengthen its relationship with residency programs in preventive medicine will serve to increase that school's involvement in public health in general. Stipends should also be available for physicians in residency programs in such fields as pediatrics, psychiatry, and medicine, to facilitate their attending a school of public health even though they are not participating in a formal residency program in preventive medicine.

Recommendations

29. *Medical schools should develop strong links with residency programs in preventive medicine and public health in their region.*

30. *To encourage the recruitment of young physicians into public health, federal support of residencies in preventive medicine and public health through schools of public health, schools of medicine, and health agencies should be stabilized at an appropriate level.*

31. *A reassessment of the status of postgraduate education in public health and preventive medicine for physicians in the clinical specialties, and in the specialty of preventive medicine is most appropriate*

at this time. The American Board of Medical Specialties should lead this review and involve the relevant medical specialty board, together with the Liaison Committee on Graduate Medical Education, the Association of American Medical Colleges, the Association of Schools of Public Health, and representatives of fields of practice.

In view of the traditional association between physicians and public health practice, it is disappointing that there is not more interchange between schools of medicine and schools of public health. In universities which have schools of medicine and public health, the latter is occasionally ignored as a teaching resource by the medical school. Conversely, not all schools of public health use existing medical school departments of physiology, or microbiology, but duplicate them. Some schools of public health originated within, or as an adjunct to, schools of medicine, and most of these have preserved a tradition of some interaction with the school of medicine on the campus.

Half the schools of medicine in the universities which also have schools of public health conduct some or most of their preventive medicine teaching through the school of public health, and several other schools of medicine are contemplating similar arrangements. Frequently, when both schools are located on the same campus, there is a system of joint faculty appointments, and they collaborate on research and community service projects. Not only do these relationships promote interaction within the academic health complex and the community, but they are also naturally helpful in developing new knowledge in public health and preventive medicine.

The Commission believes that with one or two exceptions, the full potential of this interchange has not been fully realized. Interaction and collaboration between medical schools and schools of public health should be fostered vigorously by the university administration in the interests of quality and economy.

Recommendation

32. *Where a school of public health and a school of medicine coexist in a university, the medical school should use the resources of the school of public health for teaching and collaborative research,*

and the school of public health should similarly use the biomedical
and clinical resources of the medical school.

A new pattern for medical education in public health has sometimes been proposed. This is one which calls for three parallel divisions: the basic medical sciences, the clinical sciences, and community health. This framework would appear to hold promise, but
it will clearly be some time before such a structure would be developed in many universities. However, the universities that already
have both schools of medicine and schools of public health have
the opportunity to achieve joint goals without great additional cost
or significant administrative disruption. The faculty of the school
of public health would supply the community health component
for the medical school, whereas the biologic and clinical sciences
would be provided within the school of medicine.

The most completely articulated program of this kind was recently developed, at least in concept, at the University of Toronto
(personal communications with Dr John Hastings, 1975) where
the school of public health was abolished as a separate school and
reorganized as a Division of Community Health within the medical
school, parallel in all respects to the clinical sciences and basic
medical sciences. The Division consists of the Department of Behavioral Sciences, the Department of Health Administration, and
the Department of Preventive Medicine and Biostatistics (including
Epidemiology and Environmental Health).

Responsibilities for microbiology, parisitology, and nutrition have
been assumed by the basic sciences grouping in the medical school.
The appointment of the Associate Dean for the Division of Community Health is made by a committee appointed by the University
President and not by the medical school, and the budget is an
identifiable element in the total medical school budget. Financial
and administrative problems of duplicating faculty for a school of
public health are thus avoided, and through these arrangements it
is expected that the entire university will be more readily and clearly
involved in higher education for public health. This program was
initiated in 1975. It will be several years before conclusions can be
made about its effectiveness, but the Commission feels that this
is an interesting experiment which should be observed.

In universities with no school of public health, the medical school is necessarily responsible for developing its own resources for teaching epidemiology, biostatistics, and health care organization and evaluation. Public health instruction in medical schools is centered in departments that are variously titled departments of preventive medicine, community medicine, public health and epidemiology, environmental health, or family and community medicine. If schools of public health function properly as regional resources, they should be able to supplement existing medical school arrangements, if these cannot be developed on a scale to meet the needs for expanded teaching in public health.

Columbia University School of Public Health already has relationships with a number of universities in the New York-New Jersey area. The School has met with the Association of Medical Colleges of New York and New Jersey, and offered itself as a resource to those institutions. The major interest of those schools has been in the School's M.D./M.P.H. program and one school is already participating. As regional activities of the schools of public health increase, it can be expected that more such arrangements will be developed.

Schools of Nursing

There are substantial differences between the educational qualifications and preparation needed for nurses who function clinically in public health programs and settings, and for nurses who are administrators or teachers in this field. Nursing in a public health setting is similar to other types of clinical nursing in that the nurses are concerned with individuals, patients, and families on a day-to-day basis; however, special emphasis is given to preventive medicine and public health principles, and work outside the hospital setting in community agencies.

While only a small proportion of graduates of baccalaureate programs in nursing enter public health, all students should have explicitly delineated community health nursing content and field experience as part of their educational program.

In studying the expanding and emerging diverse roles of nursing practice in response to the changing nature of the health care delivery system, the National Commission for the Study of Nursing and Nursing Education recommended a change in baccalaureate nursing education which advocates a return to specialization at the baccalaureate level. "One career pattern would emphasize nursing practice that is essentially curative and restorative . . . provided in the setting of the hospital or inpatient facility . . ." and the other " . . . distributive, would emphasize the nursing practice that is essentially designed for health maintenance and disease prevention . . . in community or emergent institutional settings." (Lysaught, 1971:90) The Commission would like to emphasize the timeliness of reconsidering specialty education at the baccalaureate level for public health nursing.

Graduate level (master's) education for public health nursing is designed to prepare:

— *administrators*: at program and agency levels; consultation, planning, and coordination functions.

—*teachers*: faculty to teach public health to nurses.

—*supervisors*: to supervise the staff nurses in clinical settings in the community; to aid in improving direct patient care services; to help build clinical nursing skills and to develop in-service education.

—*advanced clinical nurses*: for specialty practice in selected health areas or for target groups (young children, mothers, mental illness, occupational settings) (Department of Public Health Nursing, 1974).

Questions arise as to the appropriate locus of graduate education for public health nursing: should it be at schools of nursing or schools of public health; and if within schools of public health, should it be in a designated public health nursing program or part of the general health administration curriculum? The Commission believes that public health nurses who will function as administrators and educators can best be developed by schools of public health, while those whose function will be in advanced clinical practice in community settings can best be accommodated at schools of nursing.

Schools of Dentistry

Dental public health program activity within schools of dentistry
has traditionally been of low priority. In the 53 schools of dentistry
in the United States, the number of programs in preventive and
community dentistry increased from two in 1956 to 47 by 1974. Not
all of these programs have equal impact on students and faculties.
In spite of the recommendations made in 1934 by the Curriculum
Survey Committee of the American Association of Dental Schools
—that 5 percent of the curriculum time should be devoted to this
field—it was not until 1969 that an estimated level of this order
was reached. Moreover, this curriculum time is often diluted with
subjects not directly or specifically related to public health, such
as hospital dentistry, jurisprudence, the history of dentistry and practice management (Petterson and Littleton, 1971).

Postgraduate specialty programs in dental public health are
available in 18 dental schools and seven schools of public health
(American Dental Association, 1974; Block, 1974). In addition, there
are 21 residency programs in public health dentistry, 11 sponsored by
federal, state, and local health agencies, eight by dental schools, and
two by schools of public health (Council on Dental Education,
1973). In order to qualify as a specialist in public health dentistry,
a dentist must have completed master's level education at a school
of public health, as well as one year's experience in an accredited
residency program.

Residency education and field experience focus on the dental
care delivery systems and dental epidemiology, including competency in assessing dental health status indices and measurements
for controlling oral disease, and on the basic principles and skills
of preventive dentistry. In addition, the master's degree in public
health is required.

Schools of Veterinary Medicine

Veterinary medicine has been integral to public health efforts
in the United States for many years. Veterinarians are involved in
prevention of diseases transmitted by animals, particularly such

diseases as psittacosis, brucellosis, leptospirosis, rabies, and tuberculosis. They are also significantly involved in activities designed to provide safe meat and dairy products.

Although the number of veterinarians who go into full-time public health work is small, many are involved on a part-time basis in addition to their own private practices, as they assist local health departments in inspection and epidemiologic activities.

There are 19 schools of veterinary medicine in this country. Courses are offered in such public health topics as epidemiology, statistics, disease control and eradication, program management and public health administration. Postgraduate training in public health is not offered at these schools and most veterinarians receiving such training obtain it at schools of public health (personal communication with the American Veterinary Medicine Association, 1975).

It would seem essential that all veterinary medicine schools offer some training in public health, as many of their graduates are likely to participate in public health programs on a full or part-time basis.

Schools of Pharmacy

Community pharmacists have a vital role to play in the success of public health programs. Many people, particularly in the lower socioeconomic groups, seek advice about health problems from pharmacists even more than from physicians (Burton and Smith, 1970). Neighborhood pharmacists are thus in an ideal position to explain the provisions of government health programs to the elderly and the poor, to assist them in obtaining needed medical care, and, in general, to explain public health issues and programs. Pharmacists' cooperation has proved to be crucial to the success of many immunization programs. The pharmacist is also a resource for epidemiologic studies and an important participant in poison control and other programs dealing with the harmful effects of drugs.

A recent national study of education in public health at schools of pharmacy (Gibson, 1972a,b and 1973) examined the curriculum in 67 participating schools (virtually all in the nation) and tested more than 6,000 graduating seniors in two different years (1969 and 1970) for adequacy of knowledge about public health. The study concluded that while public health was taught in most but not all colleges of pharmacy, in more than half of those where it was taught, it was characterized by the school itself as unsatisfactory. There was great variation among the schools in terms of faculty and subject matter. The study recommended that each college of pharmacy review its public health teaching, that more permanent, full-time faculty specifically prepared to teach public health were needed, and that courses should be oriented towards those areas of public health most needed by the practicing pharmacist. Field work for students was recommended as an important element in the suggested required course in public health.

Schools of Optometry

A national study of optometric education in 1973 recommended that "the curriculum of schools of optometry should give greater emphasis to . . . public and community . . ." among the other areas needing strengthening (Havighurst, 1973). The Commission surveyed all 12 schools and colleges of optometry, and concluded that there is a need for more instruction in public health and community medicine. Most of the full-time faculty for these subjects have only master's level degrees from schools of public health.

Little knowledge of public health is expected from a student when he completes his academic education at a school of optometry. Public and community health is buried in the "Social, Legal, Ethical, Economic and Professional Aspects of Optometry" section of the examinations given by the National Board of Examiners in Optometry. More and more optometrists are now active in administrative planning and design of vision care programs in official health agencies.

Schools of Podiatric Medicine

The six colleges of podiatric medicine offer relatively few courses directly related to public health. However, the national boards in podiatric medicine require a demonstration of competency in community health. Podiatrists are involved in a variety of public health programs. In 1973 the American Public Health Association formally acknowledged this relationship by establishing a section in podiatric medicine. There are now 747 members enrolled (personal communication with The Membership Office, American Public Health Association, 1974).

Summary

Educational efforts in public health in the health professional schools have increased in the last two decades. However, there is no one type of professional school where the program is adequate, and all could do with some review and expansion. Greater exposure to the public health knowledge base is needed, both in the curricula of these schools and in field experience in public health for students. This exposure would provide students with positive role models in public health, and with familiarity in the community application of their own particular clinical specialty. The programs in all the health professional schools could benefit from a close relationship with a school of public health, if one is available, or with some other organized focus for higher education in public health.

Recommendation

33. The curriculum in schools of the health professions such as nursing, dentistry, veterinary medicine, pharmacy, optometry, and podiatry should be strengthened, with improved and extended instruction in the elements of the knowledge base of public health relevant to the practice of their respective professions. This should include instruction in the measurement sciences of public health, environmental health concerns, the organization, delivery and evaluation of health services, and field experience in public health programs.

12. Other Professional Schools:

Law, Engineering, Social Work, Communication and Education

Public health activities increasingly involve professionals from many different disciplines. It is essential that a firm base for collaborative efforts be established during the course of professional education, so that interpreters will not be needed when professionals from various disciplines meet in the field. Several professional schools, such as law, engineering, and social work, have already established courses and programs designed to provide their students with some knowledge of public health problems and practices. However, there is a need to develop these efforts more systematically.

Schools of Law

In recent years there has been a great increase in the amount of federal legislation relating to health; many more administrative regulations, rules, guidelines, etc., seeking to flesh out the legislation and to promote the objectives of the legislative enactments; new and modified legal doctrine coming from litigation, and the products of medical research with their opportunities and their risks. The delivery of personal medical care has essentially become a regulated industry, and regulation of many other activities that have an impact on health—such as those that affect the environment—has increased dramatically.

With the growth of legal concerns in the health field, more attorneys have become conversant with matters affecting health and human services, and there has been some increase in instruction in schools of law in regard to health matters. Thus if not now, at least soon, there will be available for almost every university community either a faculty member or a practicing attorney who devotes a large portion of time to the health field and who can provide some competent instruction on the law as it pertains to public health.

Law schools are proving to be increasingly responsive. The Commission undertook a survey of 22 large and nationally prominent law schools, and found course offerings either directly or indirectly related to public health and medical care. In addition to the more established courses in Law and Psychiatry, and Forensic Medicine, newer aspects of public health are being addressed in such courses as "Delivery of Health Care Services," "Medical Experimentation on Humans," and "Environmental Law." In addition, several institutes and research centers in health law and policy have been established, frequently in association with schools of law.

There are other methods which might acquaint law students with the health field and with the idea that there are desirable careers for them related to health. There could be a modest increase in courses related to health in law schools, options whereby law students could take courses in schools of public health, and opportunities for independent study with faculty members who have a personal interest in the health field. There has been a substantial increase in the number of cases related to health problems. A greater use of these would be one simple way of increasing the exposure of law students to public health.

Schools of Engineering

While students specializing in environmental health engineering are usually exposed to at least some phases of public health, there has been a tendency in recent years to neglect these in favor of a higher degree of engineering specialization. At the same time there is a growing need in all branches of engineering to understand the fundamentals of public health, so that engineers can adequately carry out their professional responsibilities with regard to the effect of the environment on health. It would, therefore, be highly desirable to introduce a general public health course into all engineering curricula (including environmental health engineering), which would cover social policy and the history and philosophy of public health, as well as the fundamentals of environmental protection.

Schools of Social Work

Public health and social work have traditionally shared a common social orientation and multidisciplinary approach to solving problems of community health and welfare. However, where public health is preventive in emphasis and community oriented, social work has for some time been predominantly clinical, concentrating upon individual rather than group problems. This has prompted schools of social work to develop much closer relationships with schools of medicine (especially departments of psychiatry) than with schools of public health. During the past decade however, social work has gradually begun to move closer to public health, as the broad concept of community services is being developed.

In 1973 there were 79 accredited graduate schools of social work in the United States, which enrolled more than 16,000 students and graduated 7,400 (Ripple, 1974). In addition, there were 215 baccalaureate programs affiliated with the Council on Social Work Education to prepare students for beginning level professional work. These graduate approximately 8,000 students annually.

More than 25,000 social workers are employed in health-related programs (National Center for Health Statistics, 1973d), and the vast majority of social workers will be concerned with health and medical care at some point, either on behalf of an individual client or while working with community groups. Social work is practiced in a wide variety of settings, and professionals are employed in both public and private agencies and institutions, and at the federal, state and local levels.

Public health social workers usually study at the graduate level in schools of social work, electing a major concentration in the medical care and public health area. These social workers apply their knowledge and skills in an employment setting actively engaged in health programs.

In recent years there has been a growing interaction between schools of public health and schools of social work. Both schools are increasing the number of faculty members with professional training in the other's disciplines, but joint appointments are relatively few. A variety of cross-listed courses exist, but there appear to be more social work students taking public health courses than the reverse. Joint degree programs are offered at a number of universities. Students obtain credits from both the school of social work and the school of public health, and receive their degree from the school in which they have elected their major course of study. Students may alternatively work toward both degrees concurrently through an extended training period. Increasing numbers of social work students are placed in public health agencies for field training, and some students with master's degrees in social work enter doctoral programs in public health.

As social work schools discover the knowledge base of public health, and as public health schools become aware of the knowledge and skills developed by social work, more meaningful cooperation can be anticipated through faculty interchange and joint teaching.

Schools of Communication
and Schools of Education

Communications arts are a vital part of efforts to educate the community about health. If journalists and other media specialists had some knowledge of the history and perspectives of public health, their activities could contribute significantly to raising the level of public understanding. Schools of journalism are currently contributing to the education of professionals in public health, as for example at the University of Minnesota, where the program in health education at the school of public health cross-lists two courses at the school of journalism. This kind of interchange could be expanded to include joint seminars for the two schools and discussions between public health and journalism practitioners, faculty, and students, perhaps on a regular basis.

Today, most journalists and people in the media get their medical information largely from physicians in clinical practice or clinical research. The kind of television programs and magazine stories currently featured reflect primarily the point of view of organized medicine.

Government and voluntary agencies at all levels do make attempts to inform the public and influence public opinion about policy changes and recommendations that they are making in their jurisdiction affecting health. In general, these have not been very effective. Organized medicine already recognizes the importance of participation in the political arena, and through the American Medical Association and state and local medical societies, physicians attempt to give information to people and influence their actions. Sometimes this influence is intended to change behavior related to health; often it is directed towards gaining support for the preferences of organized medicine regarding the conditions for the practice of medicine, health insurance, etc.

Teachers in the primary and secondary schools of the nation also influence public perceptions, as they lay the foundation of their students' understanding and behavior in relation to health. Students in these fields should be helped to develop an awareness of public health concerns, so that they will be able to evaluate problems with understanding. Schools of education should promote similar interactions as in journalism with educators and practitioners in public health, so as to strengthen the potential effectiveness of the teachers in the classroom in regard to public health concepts, needs, and programs.

Recommendation

34. *Graduate programs at nonhealth professional schools whose fields of practice have interfaces with public health—for example law, engineering, social work, communications, and education— should develop links with educational programs in public health in order to give their students an understanding and appreciation of public health perspectives and programs.*

References

American Academy of Family Physicians
  1974   Reprint 164 (May 2).
American Dental Association
  1974   Annual Report 1973–74: Advanced Dental Education. Chicago: American Dental Association.
American Hospital Association
  1974   Hospital Statistics. Chicago: American Hospital Association.
American Veterinary Medicine Association
  1975   Personal communication, January.
Argyris, C., and D.A. Schon
  1974   Theory in Practice: Increasing Professional Effectiveness. San Francisco: Jossey-Bass.
Association of Academic Health Centers
  1975   Personal communication, October.
Association of Schools of Allied Health Professions
  1971   Allied Health Education Programs in Senior Colleges, 1971. Compiled by contract number NIH71-4027. Department of Health, Education and Welfare publication # NIH73–241.
Association of Schools of Public Health
  1975   Data. August.
Association of State and Territorial Health Officials
  1975a   1974 Inventory Health Programs Reported by State and Territorial Health Agencies. May ASTHO–HPRS Publication #7502.
  1975b   Initial Report on Programs and Expenditures of State and Territorial Health Agencies, Fiscal Year 1974. May:13. ASTHO–HPRS Publication #7501.
Association of Teachers of Preventive Medicine
  1974   Newsletter 21 (Spring).
Biggs, H.M.
  1898   "Sanitary science, the medical profession and the public." The Medical News 67:44–50.
Block, L.
  1974   Educational Programs in Dental Public Health at Schools of

Public Health, Fall, 1973. Paper presented at American Public Health Association meeting, New Orleans, October.

Breslow, L.
1973   Statement before the House Subcommittee on Public Health and Environment, July 25.

Brockington, C.F.
1954   Quoting Simon in The Health of the Community. London: Churchill.

Bureau of Health Resources Development
1974a   Traineeships for Professional Public Health Personnel, Section 306, Public Health Science Act, Number of Trainees by Type of Program, 1957–72. Review of data sent on request (May). Washington, D.C.: Department of Health, Education and Welfare.
1974b   Grants for Residency Programs in Preventive Medicine and Dental Public Health, Annual Reports, FY68–74. Review of data sent on request (May). Washington, D.C.: Department of Health, Education and Welfare.

Burton, L.E., and H.H. Smith
1970   "The public health role of the practicing pharmacist." In Public Health and Community Medicine for the Allied Medical Professions: 516. Baltimore: Williams and Wilkins.

Cary, H.
1973   Personal communications, September (Director of Office for Membership Services, American Public Health Association, Washington, D.C.). Data reviewed from American Public Health Association membership survey as of 1973.

Chanlett, E.T.
1973   Environmental Protection. Series in Water Resources and Environmental Engineering. New York: McGraw Hill.

Commission on Education for Health Administration
1975a   Report. Vol. 1. Ann Arbor: Health Administration Press.
1975b   Ibid., p. 81.

Commission on Nontraditional Study
1973   Diversity by Design. Ed. S.B. Gould. Higher Education Series. San Francisco: Jossey-Bass.

Committee on Environmental Health Problems
1962   Report to Surgeon General, Health, Education and Welfare. United States Public Health Service, #908. Washington, D.C.: Department of Health, Education and Welfare.

Committee on Financing of Higher Education for Adult Students

1974   Financing Part-time Students: The New Majority in Post-secondary Education. A report to Office of Governmental Relations. Washington, D.C.: American Council on Education.

Committee, National Academy of Science
1966   Waste Management and Control. Publication #1400. Washington, D.C.: National Research Council.

Committee on Professional Education, American Public Health Association
1942   "Memorandum regarding minimum educational facilities for the post-graduate education of those seeking careers in public health." American Journal of Public Health 32 (May): 533–34.

Council on Dental Education
1973   Accredited Advanced Dental Education Programs. Chicago: American Dental Association (July).

Davis, K.
1975   "Equal treatment and unequal benefits: the Medicare program." Milbank Memorial Fund Quarterly/Health and Society 53 (Fall): 449–488.

Department of Public Health Nursing
1974   Public Health Nursing. Document prepared by faculty (April). Chapel Hill: School of Public Health of the University of North Carolina at Chapel Hill.

Division of Medical Education
1973   Directory of Approved Internships and Residencies, 1973–74: 3. Chicago: American Medical Association.

Dresch, S.P.
1974   An Economic Perspective on the Evaluation of Graduate Education. Technical report no. 1 to National Board of Graduate Education (March).

Englebert, E.A.
1974   "The professional competencies of public managers." Public Administration News and Views 24 (July). American Society for Public Administration.

Filerman, G.L.
1975   Personal communication, June (Executive Director, Association of University Programs in Health Administration).

Gibson, M.R.
1972a   "Public health education in colleges of pharmacy. I Background and the problems." American Journal of Pharmaceutical Education 36 (May): 189–200.
1972b   "Public health education in colleges of pharmacy. II A

survey of instruction." American Journal of Pharmaceutical Education 36 (November): 561–570.

1973   "Public health education in colleges of pharmacy. III The testing, analysis of tests, conclusions and recommendations." American Journal of Pharmaceutical Education 37 (February): 1–27.

Grove, R.D., and A.M. Hetzel
1968   Vital Statistics of the United States, 1940–1960, p. 79. United States Public Health Service Publications #1677. Washington D.C.: United States Center for Health Statistics.

Hall, T., et al.
1973a   Professional Health Manpower for Community Health Programs. Report compiled by School of Public Health of the University of North Carolina at Chapel Hill, North Carolina.

1973b   Ibid. p. 14.
1973c   Ibid. p. 20.
1973d   Ibid. p. 16.
1973e   Ibid. p. 117.

Hanft, R.
1974   Personal communication, August (Institute of Medicine, National Academy of Science).

Hanlon, J.J.
1972   "Contributions of the biological sciences to human welfare: environmental hazards." Federation Proceedings 31 (November–December): 101–120.

Hastings, J.
1975   Personal communications, September (Dean, Division of Community Health, University of Toronto, Faculty of Medicine).

Havighurst, R.J.
1973   Optometry: Education for the Profession. Report of the National Study of Optometric Education. Washington, D.C.: National Commission on Accrediting.

Hawthorne, M., and J.W. Perry
1974   Community Colleges and Primary Health Care: Study of Allied Health Education (SAHE) Report. p. iii Washington D.C.: American Association of Community and Junior Colleges.

Health Services Research Center and School of Public Health of the University of North Carolina at Chapel Hill and Milbank Memorial Fund Committee for the Study of Higher Education for Public Health

1974   1974 National Survey of Public Health Officers. Table 14. Chapel Hill, N.C.

Hibbard, P.

      Personal communications and transmitted data (Council of State Governments, Lexington, Kentucky).

Institute of Medicine

1974   Costs of Education in the Health Professions: Report of a Study. Parts I and II. Washington, D.C.: National Academy of Science.

Jain, S.C.

1975   Personal communication, August (Chairman, Department of Health Administration, School of Public Health, University of North Carolina at Chapel Hill).

Johnson, W.L.

1975   Letter of May 13 stating data as of October 1974 (Director, Division of Research, National League for Nursing, Inc.).

Katz, D., and R.L. Kahn

1966   Social Psychology of Organizations. New York: Wiley.

Klosky, J.C., ed.

1071   Register of Environmental Engineering Graduate Programs. Newark, Delaware: Association of Environmental Engineering Professors (University of Delaware).

Kraff, M.M.

1972   "Undergraduate education in hospital and health administration: dimensions and future directions." From Program Notes, No. 47 (June). Washington: Association of University Programs in Health Administration.

Lysaught, J.P., ed.

1970–71 An Abstract for Action. I:90. New York: McGraw Hill.

McLean, R.H.

1975   Personal communication, May (Bureau of Health Education, Community Program Development Division, Center for Disease Control, Region IV, Department of Health, Education and Welfare).

Magnuson, H.J.

1971   Environmental Health Activities of Schools of Public Health. Speech at Annual Meeting of Association of Schools of Public Health, May.

Membership Office, American Public Health Association

1974   Personal communication, December.

National Center for Health Statistics
  1969   Vital Statistics of the United States, 1967. Vol. II- Mortality.
            Part A. Washington, D.C: Department of Health, Education
            and Welfare.
  1973a   Health Resources Statistics: 1972–1973. Washington, D.C.:
            Department of Health, Education and Welfare.
  1973b   Ibid. p. 135.
  1973c   Ibid. p. 128.
  1973d   Ibid. p. 165.
  1973e   Ibid. p. 295.
  1974a   Monthly Vital Statistics Report: 1973–74 Nursing Home
            Survey, Provisional Data. 23 #6 Supplement, September 5.
            Washington, D.C.: Department of Health, Education and
            Welfare.
  1974b   Ibid. p. 467.
National Safety Council
  1975   Communications in January.
National Task Force on the Continuing Education Unit
  1974   The Continuing Education Unit: Criteria and Guidelines.
            Washington, D.C.: National University Extension Association.
Oakley, D.
  1973   "Population research and training in United States schools
            of public health." American Journal of Public Health 63
            (August): 657–93.
Office of Management and Budget, Statistical Policy Division
  1973   Social Indicators, 1973. Washington, D.C.: United States
            Government Printing Office.
Parran, T.
  1943–44 Public Health Schools and the Nation's Health. Dedicatory
            Address, University of Michigan: 12.
Parsons, T.
  1951   Social Structure and Dynamic Process: A Case of Modern
            Medical Practice in the Social System. Chapter 10. Glencoe,
            Illinois: Free Press.
Parsons, T., and R. Fox
  1952   "Illness, therapy and the urban family." Journal of Social
            Issues 8:31–45.
Parsons, W.B.
  1975   Personal communication, August 19.
Perrott, G. St. J.

1945   "A comprehensive training program for public health personnel." American Journal of Public Health 32 (November): 1155.

Petterson, E.O., and P.A. Littleton, Jr.
1971   "Preventive and community dentistry in the dental schools of the United States." Journal of Public Health Dentistry 31 (Fall): 256–67.

President's Science Advisory Committee, Environmental Pollution Panel
1965   Restoring The Quality of Our Environment. Report to the President (November) Washington, D.C.: The White House.

Richardson, A.H.
1973a   Report of the Fiscal Scheme Study for the Association of Schools of Public Health. Johns Hopkins University, May 5. Bureau of Manpower Education Contract NIH 71–4159.
1973b   Ibid. Table 2.

Ripple, L., ed.
1974   Statistics on Graduate Social Work Education in the United States: 1973. New York: Council on Social Work Education.

Roberts, D.E.
1068   Nurses in Public Health. Washington, D.C.: Department of Health, Education and Welfare.

Rosen, G.
1958   A History of Public Health. New York: MD Publications 468.

Rosenau, M.
1913   Progress and Problems in Preventive Medicine. Ether Day Address, Massachusetts General Hospital: 29.

Rosenfeld, L., et al.
1953   Schools of Public Health in the United States. Report based on survey of schools of public health in 1950. U.S. Public Health Service #276. Washington, D.C.: U.S. Department of Health, Education and Welfare: 29.

Saunders, C.B., Jr.
1975   Recommendations for Amendment of title IV (Student Assistance) Higher Education Act. Presentation to members of Subcommittee on Postsecondary Education, Committee on Education and Labor, United States House of Representatives. Washington, D.C: American Council on Education (Director, Office of Governmental Relations).

School of Public Health, University of Illinois
1972   Proposal for the Degree, Master of Public Health. January: 1.

School of Public Health, University of North Carolina at Chapel Hill
    1974   Public Health Nursing. April. Document prepared by the
              faculty of the Department of Public Health Nursing.
Sigerist, H.E.
    1956   Quoting Frank in Landmarks in the History of Hygiene.
              London: Oxford University Press.
Simonds, S.K.
    1975   Personal communication, May (Professor of Health Education,
              School of Public Health, University of Michigan).
Southern Regional Educational Board
    1974   Annual Report, 1973–74. Atlanta, Georgia.
Starr, S.
    1975   Personal Communications. May (Technical Services Branch,
              Division of Health Manpower and Statistics, Department of
              Health, Education and Welfare).
Sydenstricker, E.
    1935   "The changing concept of public health." Milbank Memorial
              Fund Quarterly 13:301.
Task Force on Environmental Health-Related Problems
    1967   A Strategy For a Livable Environment. A report to Secretary,
              Department of Health, Education and Welfare (June).
Terris, M.
    1973   Evolution of Public Health and Preventive Medicine in the
              United States. (Address at the Fogarty International Center
              Workshop, March 8–10 Bethesda, Maryland.)
The New York Times
    1974   (November 9).
United States Bureau of the Census
    1973   Statistical Abstract of the United States 1973. 94th Edition.
              Washington, D.C.
United States Public Health Service Act #309(a)
    1958   Hill-Rhodes Formula.
United States Public Health Service Act #309(c)
    1958   General Education Support.
Welch, W., and W. Rose
    1916a   Annual Report to Trustees of the Rockefeller Foundation
              on the Institute of Hygiene: 415.
    1916b   Ibid. p. 666.
Western Interstate Commission for Higher Education
    1972   Annual Report, 1971. Boulder, Colorado.

White, B.
  1973   Maternal and Child Health Programs in Schools of Public
           Health. October (working paper prepared for the Milbank
           Memorial Fund Commission).
White, P.E., et al.
  1974   A Survey of 1956–72 Graduates of American Schools of
           Public Health. Johns Hopkins University, December (Bureau
           of Manpower Education Contract NIH71–459).
Winkelstein, W., Jr.
  1975   Personal communication, July (Dean, School of Public Health,
           University of California at Berkeley).
Winslow, C.–E.A.
  1937   Quoting Mountin in "Report of the roundtable on the hy-
           giene aspects of housing." In New Health Frontiers: 35–45.
           Proceedings of Fifteenth Annual Conference of Milbank Me-
           morial Fund, New York.
  1948   Quoting Simon in "Poverty and disease." American Journal
           of Public Health 38:173.
World Health Organization
  1907a   The education of engineers in environmental health. Tech-
           nical Report Series 376:8. Geneva: World Health Organiza-
           tion.
  1967b   Ibid. p. 7.
  1973   "Postgraduate education and training in public health."
           Technical Report Series #533:53. Geneva:World Health
           Organization.
Wren, G.R.
  1967   Graduate education for hospital administration: a compari-
           son of Public Health and Business School Programs. Hospital
           Administration 12 (Fall):33–64.

Recommendations

The history of higher education for public health is one of unco-ordinated and often unplanned growth in response to separately perceived needs. As public health activities expanded to include new fields and new techniques, new schools, programs, and courses of instruction were created, with no overall evaluation of how these would compete with, or complement, each other. This Commission has attempted to define the desiderata of higher education in relation to current and future public health problems, to examine the educational efforts in existing institutions, and to suggest ways in which these same institutions can make a maximum contribution towards improving the health of the American people.

Constrained by reality and by the urgency of need, we have chosen to make all our recommendations applicable to existing in-stitutions and agencies. Rather than proposing new systems of education, we have begun with the existing university programs and schools, and considered how these could be made into new and more effective organizations. Great strides have been made in higher education for public health in the United States in the short time since its inception. It now remains for each school and university to consolidate and facilitate what has been achieved in the past, so that the superseding goal of protecting, promoting, and restoring the people's health can be reached.

The recommendations of the Commission for restructuring higher education for public health are listed below in the order in which they appear in the report. A full discussion, explaining the Com-mission's reasoning for these recommendations, will be found in the text in the chapters noted after each recommendation.

Recapitulation of Recommendations

1. A concerted national effort should be undertaken to develop a larger and better qualified cadre of professional personnel capable of coping with the complex and changing health problems of the

nation. Because higher education for public health is a national concern, the responsibility for this endeavor should be shared by federal and state governments, educational institutions and operating health agencies. (Chapter 3: Public Health Activities and Organizations)

2. A national program to monitor systematically the needs for, and supply of, public health manpower is crucial to effective planning of education for the field. Such a program should be developed and conducted by the Department of Health, Education, and Welfare, in continuous cooperation with universities, relevant professional organizations, and public health agencies. (Chapter 4: Personnel for Public Health)

3. In order to produce professional personnel with appropriate knowledge, skills, and perspective so that they might deal effectively with the new challenges in public health, all institutions providing higher education for public health should build their educational programs on the unique knowledge base for public health. This combines the three elements central and generic to public health with content from many related fields such as medicine and other patient care disciplines; economics, political science, and sociology; biology and the physical sciences. The elements central to public health are the measurement and analytic sciences of epidemiology and biostatistics; social policy and the history and philosophy of public health; and the principles of management and organization for public health. This knowledge base may be modified and expanded with changes in the nature and scope of health problems and the techniques used to deal with them, but an appropriate mix of its central elements with selected related fields is crucial to the effectiveness of any program of higher education for public health. (Chapter 5: The Knowledge Base for Public Health)

4. There should be a major redirection and reorganization of higher education for public health, based on the recognition that different groups of personnel with different functions will require different kinds of educational programs.
A. The schools of public health should concentrate their efforts primarily on:

    (1) The preparation of people who will function as executives, planners, and policy-makers.

    (2) The preparation of epidemiologists and biostatisticians.

    (3) The preparation of research scientists and educators.

B. Individual graduate programs in other schools in universities should continue concentrating on the preparation of people who will function at the operating level in respective specialty fields of public health. (Chapter 7: A Rational Structure)

5. Each school of public health should develop a clear statement of its educational mission, and the plan that it has developed for the preparation of personnel for executive and leadership roles in public health in general, and in the specialties of public health practice, the training of epidemiologists, biostatisticians, research scientists, and educators. This statement must have the concurrence and support of the university administration. (Chapter 8: The Schools of Public Health)

6. The schools of public health should provide technical assistance for the growing number of programs in other parts of the university which train certain types of manpower for the field. They should serve as regional resources to consult and participate in academic planning with all graduate programs in higher education for public health within specified geographic areas. (Chapter 8: The Schools of Public Health)

7. Federal and state governments should provide financial support which will enable and encourage schools of public health to fulfill important functions as regional resources for the production of appropriately trained manpower for public health. (Chapter 8: The Schools of Public Health)

8. Schools of public health should require that before admission to their program of training for executive and leadership functions, students have either:

    (1) A professional degree in one of the health professions.

    (2) A graduate degree in a field relevant to public health.

    (3) A minimum of three years' experience in a public health program.

Entering students should have an adequate knowledge of the bio-logic basis of health problems, and the basic concepts of social and behavioral sciences so that they can understand the background of the economic, social, and political aspects of public health, or schools should plan for, and ensure that, necessary compensatory courses are provided early in the student's educational program. (Chapter 8: The Schools of Public Health)

9. In order to overcome the isolation of faculty compartmentaliza-tion, the faculty of schools of public health should be organized so that related skills and knowledge are unified for teaching and re-search. (Chapter 8: The Schools of Public Health)

10. In order to ensure high quality and to avoid unnecessary dupli-cation of faculty, the university administration should support and facilitate intrauniversity arrangements which would enable depart-ments in the social, management, and biomedical sciences to work together with faculty in schools of public health wherever this would contribute effectively to meeting the education and research needs of the school. (Chapter 8: The Schools of Public Health)

11. Project grants to meet national needs for specific kinds of public health manpower should be targeted and time-limited for those pur-poses so that they do not encourage the unnecessary development of permanent programs. Schools should adapt to these short-term needs where they can without altering their long-term objectives. (Chapter 8: The Schools of Public Health)

12. To protect and support high standards, and to avoid costly com-petition and duplication of resources, all schools of public health should recognize that certain schools have particular strengths in specialized areas, and are national centers of excellence. Thus, doc-toral training and research in these fields should be concentrated at these centers. (Chapter 8: The Schools of Public Health)

13. Supervised programs of field experience in connection with aca-demic activity must be an integral and significant part of education for public health responsibility. (Chapter 8: The Schools of Public Health)

14. Faculty members in schools of public health should undertake periodic, if not continuous, formal responsibilities in the operation of community health services which are relevant to, and will be supportive of, their respective fields of academic responsibility. (Chapter 8: The Schools of Public Health)

15. Educational institutions should develop reciprocal relationships with health agencies and community organizations to bring greater realism to the classroom, and academic expertise to the field. They should also solicit, and be responsive to, evaluations of their educational programs provided by these agencies. (Chapter 8: The Schools of Public Health)

16. Recognized centers at American schools of public health should continue to train foreign nationals in those areas of specialization for which appropriate education is not available in their home or other nearby countries. These centers should also carry out a systematic program of faculty exchange and collaborative research with foreign institutions. (Chapter 8: The Schools of Public Health)

17. Programs for the training of foreign nationals should give adequate consideration to the particular cultural, organizational, and socioeconomic needs of the individual student and/or nation. (Chapter 8: The Schools of Public Health)

18. Universities that have, or are establishing, programs designed to prepare people for public health activity, should establish an administrative focus at the highest level, next to the President, for planning and development, so as to ensure that all relevant elements of the knowledge base are appropriately represented through optimum use of university resources. (Chapter 9: Individual Programs in Public Health Fields)

19. All programs of higher education for public health should have close relationships with the field of practice similar to those recommended for schools of public health, and faculty in these programs should have similar field and advocacy responsibilities. (Chapter 9: Individual Programs in Public Health Fields)

20. Federal, state, and institutional aid must be made available for minority groups and other students with substantial financial needs in order to ensure equity of access to education for public health. (Chapter 10: Special Responsibilities and Problems)

21. In all institutions providing higher education for public health, continuing education should occupy a distinct and prominent role in the program:
    (1) There should be a clearly defined focus of responsibility for academic and administrative components.
    (2) Coherent programs should be developed to fill identified gaps in knowledge for target groups of professionals.
    (3) Basic standardized national criteria should be developed to ensure quality of course offerings, and to facilitate the systematic recording of individual and institutional participation in programs of continuing education. (Chapter 10: Special Responsibilities and Problems)

22. Educational institutions preparing people for public health should expect faculty members to serve as informed advocates of effective health policies, programs, and practices, and firmly support them even if such advocacy becomes controversial. (Chapter 10: Special Responsibilities and Problems)

23. A sustained and heightened research effort is needed in all graduate programs providing higher education for public health. The schools of public health have special opportunities to focus their unique interdisciplinary perspective and resources on the development of research, both applied and basic, on a wide range of present and emerging public health problems. (Chapter 10: Special Responsibilities and Problems)

24. There is a distinct and continuous national need for people who will function as executives, planners, policy-makers and leaders in the field of public health, epidemiologists, biostatisticians, research scientists, and educators. Therefore, the schools of public health should receive continuous basic support from the federal govern-

ment to carry out educational programs to satisfy this need. (Chapter 10: Special Responsibilities and Problems)

25. State governments should provide—as some do now—financial support for all graduate programs which prepare people for public health activity at the operating level in state and local public health programs. (Chapter 10: Special Responsibilities and Problems)

26. Academic institutions responding to national needs for specific types of public health manpower should receive federal grant support for that purpose. This support, should, of course, be time-limited where this is appropriate in terms of the estimate of national need. (Chapter 10: Special Responsibilities and Problems)

27. Because a medical education will continue to provide many professionals with a basic foundation for important responsibilities in public health, medical schools should provide more emphasis on such subjects as epidemiology, preventive medicine, the organization, delivery, and evaluation of health care, and environmental health concerns. (Chapter 11: Related Professional Schools)

28. The current status of the teaching of community health in medical schools should be reviewed, and strong positive programs to correct deficiencies should be developed. The Association of American Medical Colleges should take the leadership for this review together with other organizations such as the Association of Schools of Public Health, the Association of Teachers of Preventive Medicine, the Association of Academic Health Centers, the American Board of Preventive Medicine, and the American College of Preventive Medicine. (Chapter 11: Related Professional Schools)

29. Medical schools should develop strong links with residency programs in preventive medicine and public health in their region. (Chapter 11: Related Professional Schools)

30. To encourage the recruitment of young physicians into public health, federal support of residencies in preventive medicine and public health through schools of public health, schools of medicine,

and health agencies should be stabilized at an appropriate level. (Chapter 11: Related Professional Schools)

31. A reassessment of the status of postgraduate education in public health and preventive medicine for physicians in the clinical specialties, and in the specialty of preventive medicine is most appropriate at this time. The American Board of Medical Specialties should lead this review, and involve the relevant medical specialty board, together with the Liaison Committee on Graduate Medical Education, the Association of American Medical Colleges, the Association of Schools of Public Health, and representatives of fields of practice. (Chapter 11: Related Professional Schools)

32. Where a school of public health and a school of medicine co-exist in a university, the medical school should use the resources of the school of public health for teaching and collaborative research, and the school of public health should similarly use the biomedical and clinical resources of the medical school. (Chapter 11: Related Professional Schools)

33. The curriculum in schools of the health professions such as nursing, dentistry, veterinary medicine, pharmacy, optometry, and podiatry should be strengthened with improved and extended instruction in the elements of the knowledge base of public health relevant to the practice of their respective professions. This should include instruction in the measurement sciences of public health, environmental health concerns, the organization, delivery, and evaluation of health services, and field experience in public health programs. (Chapter 11: Related Professional Schools)

34. Graduate programs at nonhealth professional schools whose fields of practice have interfaces with public health—for example law, engineering, social work, communications and education—should develop links with educational programs in public health in order to give their students an understanding and appreciation of public health perspectives and programs. (Chapter 12: Other Professional Schools)

Postword

When the report of the Commission was being drafted, several members expressed the need for some concluding comments. They believed that the breadth of considerations and intensity of discussions could not readily be summarized in a text of manageable proportions. The Chairman, ex officio, was entrusted with writing further thoughts on both the work of the Commission and the content of its report. These comments are intended as neither an apologia nor a concluding statement, but rather as the Chairman's reflection upon the importance of *continuing* the critical assessments and interim judgments made herein.

The general national context within which the Commission's work was undertaken in 1972 changed in many significant ways in the intervening years. *Higher education* and *public health* have not escaped the impact of economic recession, loss of confidence in the efficiency of government programs, or the accountability of public regulatory mechanisms. For example, the probability of a "steady-state" in the financing of higher education apparent in 1972, became the actuality of "selective cutbacks" by 1975. The mirage of increased public policy commitments to ensure accessibility of health services receded on the horizon. And the interdependence of collective action and personal responsibility in the maintenance of health and prevention of disease has become obscured in the increased attention given to life style.

Notwithstanding these changes in the nation—and their implication for civil liberties, social justice, and economic strength are no less profound than for health—the Commission has dealt squarely with the abiding question within its charge, i.e. higher education for public health. The very changes which have loomed large in the two sectors make the more circumscribed yet overriding focus of the Commission's task even more relevant. The need for effective education for professionals to help them in understanding these changes, and for vigorous leadership in guiding public policy to accommodate them, has never been greater.

In facing the future programming of education activities to prepare more and better professional personnel for the immediate and long-term future, more money to support all efforts in higher education for public health, as currently conducted, would clearly not, by itself, meet the challenge. Thus, the need for review and assessment of current programs, and planning for some change seems clear. There is a great need to enhance the problem-solving capacity of our society in many areas, including the field of public health. As demands are being made upon universities to deal more directly with society's problems, their activities are being subjected to more scrutiny, criticism, and influence. Universities have become dependent on federal funds for basic financing, the dollar value of which has increased as has the ratio of this contribution to the total resources of the institutions. The latter are discomfited that the intellectual resources that society has traditionally, and often passively, expected to be harnessed in its service are now being more specifically demanded in return for this fiscal support. As Henry Sigerist said some 30 years ago; "Universities are like beautiful women. They like to be admired but not discussed."

The increasing appreciation of the need for science and for technological understanding on the part of our society inevitably focuses attention on the universities of the nation more than ever before. The discomfort of being scrutinized should be welcomed because it is an antidote to the natural tendency of faculty members to be most comfortable doing what they've done before, particularly after they have obtained tenure and the approbation of their peers.

The effectiveness of university responses, and the appropriateness of society's expectations, will ultimately be measured not just by the magnitude of budgets or by the size of student enrollments. The quality of direct faculty involvement in the field, and the performance of professional responsibilities by graduates, will surely enter into any long-range validation.

The Commission has described the development of different types of university programs of education for public health. A striking feature is the absence of a specific framework of structure, function, and process among these programs. Respecting this diversity, we developed a basic formulation that would, however, rationalize the current system and at the same time improve it.

It was not our intention to recommend an inflexible pattern for future development. The specificity of our recommendations— though they appear logical to the Commission—does not mean that there may not be other, perhaps better, ways of achieving the objectives that we outlined. However, a rational, organized approach to the framework of preparing the range of professional personnel needed for public health today is vital. We are not opposed to pluralism, but what exists now is chaotic, wasteful, and dysfunctional. What is needed is greater clarity of purpose to serve urgent public need. We have developed what we believe is a rational approach to university-wide responsibility in this field, and have indicated ways in which different universities can determine and carry out roles appropriate to their resources and their missions.

The recommendations regarding the importance of developing special education programs to prepare people for leadership positions may be labeled by a few as "elitist." Any connotation of exclusivity of entry is not intended by the Commission. The recommendation aims only to recognize that the complexity of public health activities requires a cadre of highly skilled people, and that people earn leadership positions through diverse pathways of work and study.

Public health work is not carried out by a single type of professional, nor does it call for a single level of activity and responsibility. The need for different mixes and levels of training is vital to every society and complex organization. However, free societies and viable organizations must assure structural opportunities to enhance one's capabilities to move to higher levels of operation. It is the differentiation between these needs and the appropriateness of educational responses which are not adequately addressed by our universities. As enrollment has increased and the number of educational programs has grown, these issues have been set aside and neglected. As a result, the stated objectives of many of the programs tend to be unrealistic and deceptive.

Manpower requirements for public health, like other areas of health services, are difficult to predict with any precision. In the absence of a national program for the monitoring and surveillance of public health personnel, the burden of manpower planning falls on the separate universities. The Commission's recommendations, if adopted in their general intent, would result in substantial change in the perceptions of need for personnel and types of educational programs. At present it would seem best to plan within the existing constellation of resources, and to improve their relevance and effectiveness rather than create new ones. This does not mean that special needs in specialized fields are to be ignored, nor should it preclude the development of consortium arrangements among colleges and universities in a region, to be responsive to such needs.

Two interrelated recommendations might be overlooked by the hurried reader as self-evident and interpreted by others as unwise and dangerous. They are the recommendations dealing with greater field involvement for faculty and students, and with strong advocacy roles for faculty members. I suggest that these are at the heart of the reforms needed. The emphasis on relating theory to practice and practice to theory is not an anti-intellectual approach to education, nor is it an attempt to intellectualize the "practical world." Perhaps the observation made by William H. McGuffey (President of Cincinnati College and author of *McGuffey's Eclectic Readers*) in 1835 is the best synthesis: "Theory, without practice, will be mischievous; and practice, without theory, must, of course, be at random. . . ." That McGuffey's postulates can be reversed merely underscores the essential nature of the two. One can never be a substitute for the other.

Our recommendation of a strong advocacy role for faculty members may cause disquiet in some quarters. But academic freedom, like all liberties, is bound to atrophy unless exercised. I believe that public health faculty members have a right and a responsibility to make contributions to public understanding of issues and policies. Society, for its part, has a right to expect that scientific knowledge will be fully harnessed in public service. Informed advocacy is not "reform-mongering," but rather an integral part of public health's commitment to enhancing the ability of an informed citizenry to formulate enlightened public policy.

In conclusion, I would like to add a brief note about the final report. All members of the Commission agreed to the recommendations, and reviewed and commented upon the penultimate draft of the text. Editorial changes have been made since then. For these attempts at clarity and economy, and for omissions and errors, responsibility rests with the Chairman and the Study Director. I cannot close these comments without expressing my most grateful appreciation for the insightful, understanding manner in which the President and staff of the Milbank Memorial Fund have helped me and my colleagues carry out our task.

CECIL G. SHEPS

Personal Statement

Ernest M. Gruenberg

The Commission's recommendations, if carried out, will not prepare us adequately for the future. Something additional is needed.

What should be the heart of the report is buried on page 59.

> "Unity is to be found rather in the ends to be accomplished— the preservation and improvement of health—than in the means essential to that end." (Welch and Rose Report, 1916a:415).

That report led to the first schools of public health; full-time departments of public health with professionally trained staffs soon became standard parts of government. The purpose unifying these establishments was the preservation of the people's health. While the essential means changed with advancing techniques, new living arrangements and styles, industrial and social innovations, and the changing patterns of disease, this end remained unchanged.

I fear that the established public health agencies (both government and voluntary) have lost that perspective as their guiding principle. It is the wide variety of means which at one time were more or less relevant to the ends to be accomplished which have become institutionalized, rather than the primary mission—to protect health. The public health schools' efforts to provide personnel for public health agencies have undermined their ability to keep central the goal of protecting the people's health.

Our report becomes so involved in saying something relevant about each of the various means currently used in public health agencies, and the wide variety of schooling sequences needed to produce people with the entire set of skills employed, that the reader can easily lose sight of the important end for which these means were devised—the *protection* of health. A reader could also get the notion that organizational and administrative skill in weaving these heterogeneous threads together into a functioning apparatus is the primary goal of health work. But if Welch and Rose were correct, as I believe they were, then the central issue is the preservation of the people's health rather than that of the health of organizations or institutions.

What, then, is the basic science of work devoted to preserving health? Some reputable leaders have answered "public health administration" and its related arts and sciences. Others agree with me that, because the goal of health work is to protect health, such work seeks to change the way diseases occur in populations by trying to postpone death and to lower the frequency with which preventable diseases and injuries occur; hence, the health movement must be guided by an epidemiologic perspective so that progress is gauged by the people's improved health.

We have often had victories in prolonging life and in lowering the prevalence rates of certain diseases (and disease-produced disabilities and miseries). These are the only true signals of success. This perspective should inform all health work and education for professionals who are preparing to function as leaders in society's organized struggles to improve health.

It is not easy to maintain that perspective. The report itself shows how hard it is to do so consistently if one gives equal weight to each of the activities which have become attached to public health agencies.

There was a time when death and disease were seen as part of human destiny, of fate—as inevitable consequences of life. This fatalism gradually yielded to the notion that certain deaths and certain diseases could be avoided. By 1916 some leaders recognized that the techniques for avoiding certain types of deaths and certain specific diseases were sufficiently advanced to justify their systematic social application by means of established units of government. It was also seen that an institute of hygiene, designed to advance knowledge and to better these techniques, could act as a center for the education of professional leaders to head these government agencies. So the actions which flowed from the 1916 Welch and Rose Report, which is the antecedent of this Commission, ended the era in which the fatalistic view prevailed. In the 30 years that followed there was a radical transformation of mortality and morbidity patterns; so the report expressed an accurate vision of the future.

I believe we are again entering a new era, as events have overtaken the institutions which emerged, and they no longer represent a vision of the future. I would guess that it is the explosion of science and technology in the last three or four decades which chiefly created the new conditions. Technical advances are occurring at an ever-accelerating rate. Society's institutions in general become less and less capable of guiding the advance of technology and the implementation of new techniques so as to better rather than to endanger human lives. The public health agencies—whether operational or educational—play an ever-decreasing role in pacing technical advances and in determining their application so as to improve people's health. New knowledge and new techniques arise in an enormous number of different settings. No one can keep up with all of them any longer. No agency is geared to monitor these advances and to estimaate their potential good or bad effects on people's health.

Disease control techniques have produced a new set of issues because they produce unplanned-for types of power: for example, we can now make filthy water safe and thus abet the process of environmental pollution. We can also prevent death without curing the underlying cause, thereby increasing the average duration of cases with certain diseases and chronic disabilities.

Even after new substances have become commonplace in the environment, there is no agency responsible for estimating their effect on the people's health. The National Center for Health Statistics was given this type of mission when it was created, but it has never had the capability of providing information on what conditions of ill health are becoming more important and which less important. So it cannot provide the information needed to guide health policies and priorities.

Technical advances are largely uncontrolled today just as disease and death were largely uncontrolled two centuries ago. Just as the patterns of disease and death have come under partial control through appropriate social institutions, using the established knowledge about modifiable factors which produce disease, so I think we are approaching a period when social planning will begin to influence and control the advances of science and technology. For example, it should not have taken a generation to recognize that new drugs would indefinitely prolong the life of mongoloid infants without improving their ability to function, so that this condition became three or four times more prevalent within a few decades. Even after that fact was demonstrated, no agency was responsible for increasing the planning of services for mongoloid adults accordingly or of assigning research resources to find a preventable cause of mongolism.

Where is the intelligence arm of the health movement now? Where will it be in the future? The epidemiologists and biostatisticians who did this so well for a period have become victims of their own advancing technology and specialization, becoming sharper and sharper at identifying more and more obscure issues while the big changes in people's health get less and less attention.

The rate of technical innovation in industry and the health-related research establishments has outstripped the ability of the agencies organized in the name of public health to provide organizational centers for priority-setting and for identifying soluble problems in the effort to preserve health. They are unable to mobilize the resources needed to solve these problems.

I believe that the agencies organized in the name of public health have become too preoccupied with maintaining the activities they struggled to create, have too many personal service missions and have already lost such a large part of their leading roles in the struggle to improve health, that we are wrong to rely exclusively upon them in the future. Just as something new was needed in 1916, so something new is needed in 1976.

A social institution whose central preoccupation is protecting *or* preserving *the people's health could examine every new technical discovery and social policy to weigh its potential impact on the people's health. It could preserve the record of past successes and failures to better the people's health, and continually reappraise the lessons to be learned from this accumulating experience.*

Higher Education for Public Health

Perhaps some schools of public health could develop postgraduate departments which embody this mission. But it is also possible that none of them can escape sufficiently from their expanded missions to perform such a feat. Perhaps the universities which acted as homes for the institutes which filled these roles for 30 years have lost their ability to provide that hospitality.

On the one hand a university faculty member should have the right to advocate public acceptance of his individual views; on the other, the necessary kind of organization should gain credibility by consistently expressing the consensus of the best available expert opinion. It is difficult to see how the two can be reconciled.

One cannot tell whether any existing schools of public health will want to try to create such a center; no one can foresee the possibilities of success until some try. I do not think we should wait to find out before recognizing that in 1976 we need to innovate again to create an institution, independently endowed, which can embody the art of formulating techniques and policies which protect the people's health. Such an institution could also provide the educational opportunities needed for higher level professionals in that kind of preventive health work.

I believe the need is apparent. I doubt that any university can provide the base for such an institution. I think it obvious that today government cannot institutionalize this value system. Whether the time is ripe for any such institution's creation I cannot judge; I only know that there is a pressing need.

This personal statement is filed with all due respect for my fellow Commissioners, the Chairman, and the staff whose discussion at Commission meetings have been responsible for leading me to these conclusions. But the conclusions recorded here were never sufficiently formulated to become a topic of Commission debate, so I do not know how pleased or shocked any of them will be or even if they will regard this suggestion as relevant. Of course, nothing I have written here can be construed as disagreement with any specific part of any of the Commission's recommendations.